Nail Q&A Book

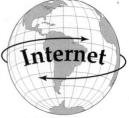

SalonOvations'
Nail Q&A Book

by

Vicki Peters

Milady Publishing
(a division of Delmar Publishers)
3 Columbia Circle, Box 2519
Albany, New York 12215

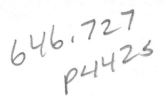

NOTICE TO THE READER

Cover Design: Suzanne Nelson

Milady Staff
Publisher: Catherine Frangie
Acquisitions Editor: Marlene McHugh Pratt
Project Editor: Annette Downs Danaher
Production Manager: Brian Yacur
Production and Art/Design Coordinator: Suzanne Nelson

COPYRIGHT © 1996
Milady Publishing
(a division of Delmar Publishers)

an *International Thomson Publishing company* I(T)P
Printed in the United States of America
Printed and distributed simultaneously in Canada

For more information, contact:
SalonOvations
Milady Publishing
3 Columbia Circle , Box 12519
Albany, New York   12212-2519

Library of Congress Cataloging-in-Publication Data

Peters, Vicki.
     SalonOvations' nail Q & A book / by Vicki Peters.
        p.   cm.
     Includes bibliographical references and index.
     ISBN: 1-56253-266-9
     1. Manicuring. I. Title
TT958.3.P48 1996
646.7'27–dc20

95-48220
CIP

This book is dedicated to my mother,
Cynthia Peters Cantwell, who lost her life
to cancer in 1989 and never lived to see
my success. I know in my heart
she is watching me now.

Contents

PART TWO

The Technical Side

Acknowledgments

Reflecting back on those who helped me along the way, brings to mind several people who influenced my career and personal development and led me to write this book.

In 1985, I met Norm Freed who continues to influence me personally and professionally. I am truly proud to be part of his "business family" and will continue to aspire to his level of understanding of the beauty industry. He made me realize that I do have something to contribute. Thank you, Norm.

I would also like to thank Paula Gilmore, the businesswoman/nail technician we should all aspire to. Her professionalism, craft, and love for this industry have been inspiring to watch. It was Paula who signed me up for my first nail competition that got my career out from behind the manicuring table. So this is all her fault! Thank you, Ms. P.

Deborah Carver, publisher of *NailPro Magazine* and Linda Lewis, executive editor: a special thank you to both these women for recognizing my desire to be a role model in this industry and helping me make it happen. The care and desire to bring good information to their pages is truly a collective passion, and I am glad to be part of their team. Thank you both for sharing my passion for the nail industry and recognizing what others did not.

Barbara Hehir, my 7th grade art teacher screams with delight every time I phone her. She is so proud of me and always knew I would succeed, well before I knew. Her continued support and understanding over the years have been a great foundation for me. Thank you, Mrs. Hehir.

I would also like to thank Tim Farquhar of Dayton, Ohio; Sheryl Macauley of Bakersfield, CA; Cris Haubruge of Mohave, CA; Anita Lime of Albany, GA; Peg Ostby from Creative Cruises; and of course, my dear friend Jewell, and all the thousands of nail techs out there who give me much more than I could ever give back. You motivate me to do more. Thanks. You are all my trophies.

I also received assistance in compiling technically accurate information for this book from some industry experts, whom I'd like to acknowledge: Douglas Schoon, chemist and author of *HIV/AIDS: Everything You Need to Know to Protect Yourself and Others*; Dr. Godfrey Mix of Rx Productions; Brian Eriksson of Aseptico; Jane Schiff; and Kristy Wells.

Also, a special thank you to the following professionals for their time and expertise in reviewing this manuscript: Stella Niffenegger, Cincinnati, OH; Joanne Wiggins, Philadelphia, PA; Barrie Allen, North Brentwood, NY; and Elizabeth Anthony, Palatine, IL.

About the Author

Vicki Peters has been a practicing licensed nail technician in California since 1982. She is a leading authority in nail competitions. Vicki spent five years managing the Nails Magazine Shows, developed Nails National Tour, and currently co-produces NailPro's Nail Institute with *NailPro Magazine.* She is a contributing editor to *NailPro,* Britain's *LNE Nouvelle Nails,* and *Health & Beauty's Nail News,* as well as a cover artist and educator. Vicki has served on the Nail Manufacturer's council and is president of her own consulting company, The Peters Perspective, in southern California.

Introduction

The positive reinforcement one gets from teaching is the most rewarding pleasure any educator can experience. I feel lucky because I now make my living teaching thousands of novice and professional nail technicians all over the world, and get this reinforcement regularly. But what my students don't realize is that I am really the student here. It is I have who have benefited most from their ideas and techniques.

That information and those techniques can be found on these pages. Years of practice, knowledge and wisdom gives you experience. This book has been written to give you that experience; to assist you in developing your career as a nail technician by understanding the basics of nail technology without product endorsements.

It seems that we often learn only enough to pass our state boards in school. Once in a while we are blessed with instructors who have a passion for this industry and care enough to share their experiences. Otherwise, we are sent out into that big world of manicuring too green to make a living. Some of us fail and some of us excel. As I have said before, I truly believe that our education begins the moment we walk out the door of beauty school. So now what? Where do we get good sound information and the technical knowledge that takes years for us to accumulate by working in salons and practicing on clients. How do we bridge the gap between inexperience and experience?

Hopefully this book will help.

PART ONE

The Business of Nails

Business Basics

Your Professional Responsibility

Q 1. What is my professional responsibility?

A To act as a true business person and take responsibility for your services. That may mean that you are at fault if the service wasn't the best. However, providing good service at all times should be a priority.

Q 2. What are professional business ethics?

A Professional business ethics is knowing how to conduct yourself and your business in a professional manner. This means greeting your clients properly and treating them well, handling your conversation politely, and knowing when and when not to talk. Providing a sanitary work environment, keeping records and staying up to date on new products and techniques is also important.

- Attire is extremely important, and remember, you mirror your clients. You tend to attract clients like yourself.
- Always have your hair, makeup, and nails done.
- Control your personal opinions and feelings, and let the client dictate the conversation.

- Greet every client and do not talk about clients after they leave.
- Be punctual at all times.
- Be conscious of your posture and make an effort to sit correctly while you are working.
- Take pride in your work.
- Never criticize the salon you work in or the other technicians and their work. It is a poor reflection on you.

Client Cards

Q *3. What information do I need on client cards?*

A Client name, address, phone number, beeper number, car phone number, date when client started coming to you, birth date, referral name, favorite polish colors, description of services, allergies, special notes and problems, recommended home care, suggested retail products, best appointment times, service fees, and the technician's initials.

Q *4. What are the benefits of keeping client cards?*

A One of the main benefits of client cards is that all the information can be accessed by another technician if you are not available. Documenting problems and products is very important. Addresses and phone numbers can be valuable if you need to do a mailing.

Q *5. Where do I get client cards?*

A Several companies in the industry offer client cards with filing boxes or small binders. Check the trade magazines for special books that list the industry's manufacturers.

Q *6. How do I file the cards?*

A File the cards by first name. We don't always remember clients' last names, and it will be easier to find their cards.

Q *7. What if I want to design my own client cards?*

A A simple word processing program will allow you to design the card you need. Photocopy the information on to a card stock. Cut it into the desired card size, or use basic 5" × 7" card stock. Use a different color for each tech in the shop to identify whose client she is. Start off each year with a new color identifying how long someone has been a client.

Q *8. How should I keep my client cards updated?*

A Each time you see the client for a repair or appointment, document the date, the service she received, and the polish color that she wore. Note purchases and home care.

Power Prescribing

Q *9. What is power prescribing?*

A Power prescribing is an assessment of the client needs. At her first appointment, schedule a few extra minutes to ask the following questions to determine her needs. Or have her come in for a consultation before her appointment.

- Why does she want nails?
- What does she want to accomplish by having nails?
- Is she ready for the commitment of having artificial nails? Explain the maintenance.

- What length does she want to wear them?
- Ask her about her lifestyle. Is she a truck driver, home-maker, business executive, or ballet dancer?
- Does she have any concerns about damaging her nails? Explain what each procedure will do to her nails.
- Would she eventually like to grow her own nails out? Does she need just a little added support or would she like full extensions?

After assessing this information, it is up to you to determine which service suits her the best. If she is a truck driver, you are not going to put long and beautifully thin fiberglass nails on her. Instead you will use a stronger service such as an acrylic tip and overlay for her.

Q *10. How can my clients benefit from power prescribing?*

A Both you and your clients benefit from prescribing the correct service in maintenance, repair, and workable nails. If you prescribe the wrong service, it will show in her nails. The wrong service will become obvious to both of you.

Q *11. What services should I prescribe?*

A You should offer every service that is available. Sculptured nails, acrylic tip and overlays, fiberglass, and gels in addition to natural nail care and natural nail overlays. If you choose to specialize in one service, then do one service well. However, you will be giving your clients only one option. If your clients wish to change services, they will need to change technicians to accomplish that.

Q *12. What kind of maintenance should I be prescribing?*

A As the technician, you need to educate your clients as to the commitment they need to make to maintain their nails properly. Artificial services such as acrylic, gel, or fiberglass will last an average of two weeks. If your client has a problem, a one week or ten day fill-in is recommended.

If you have a client with slow growing nails or one who is easy on her nails, suggest she go three weeks or more without any service. And remember, clients should be serviced prior to experiencing problems in order to maintain optimal natural nail health!

Schedule a complimentary "touch up" appointment at the 7- to 10-day mark after applying a full set to any new client. Intercepting any premature lifting, reshaping the nails, or taking the length down will make the client comfortable and secure her loyalty.

Q 13. Can I guarantee my work?

A There are no guarantees in life—just warranties. You can comfortably warranty your work as long as you give clear parameters. Below is an example. Make your own guidelines and put them in writing.

Example:

Offer a 14-day warranty with the provision that she use cuticle oil every day and wear gloves when gardening and doing dishes. If the nails still break, offer to repair them free of charge.

Q 14. What do I do when the service I prescribed doesn't work?

A Try an alternative option. Not all services work on all clients. Test it on one nail before changing over completely. Test nails should be applied 24 hours prior to applying the full set in order to avoid/detect possible problems (such as allergies or chemical reactions).

Most important, try to identify if there is a problem with your work. Don't be defensive. Look to see if you need to make them thicker. Check the sides or try a different product.

If you cannot define what the problem is, have another technician look at the nails for you. Do not discuss the problem in front of the client. Take it to the back room after she leaves. There is usually an answer and sometimes it takes another technician to see it. Identifying the problem is your responsibility and yours to correct, however you may find it.

Q 15. *Should I follow up on my clients?*

A Yes! A new full-set client should always get a follow-up call from the technician two to three days after her appointment. Intercepting any problems ahead of time can save an unhappy client and secure one that is.

If you are not comfortable making the call (none of us like rejection) have your salon owner make the call. If for some reason the client is unhappy, the salon owner needs to understand why so she can help the technician improve. If the client is happy with your services, it is also important that the salon owner is aware of how well you are servicing your clients.

Q 16. *How should I follow up?*

A Have a written questionnaire ready if you are going to make a call. Ask the client if it is a good time to talk about her nails. Be sure to have a place on the top of the questionnaire for the client's name and date.

Start by identifying yourself and the purpose of the call. Ask:

- How is she doing with her new nails?
- If they are too long does she need to come in for a shortening?
- Does she like the shape?
- Are there any problems (such as lifting)?
- Was she happy with the services she received?
- Confirm or schedule the next appointment!

Another option is to put a thank you note in the mail along with a questionnaire and a stamped, self-addressed return envelope. You can ask for more detailed information that way.

Q *17. What if the client is not happy with my service?*

A This can be an awkward situation but one that can be handled well. The bottom line is to keep the client coming to the salon. You do not want to lose the client to another salon. Ask her what you can do to rectify the problem and suggest placing her with another technician. Make the client feel as comfortable as possible when she returns to the salon. Identify and correct the problem as best you can.

Record Keeping

Q *18. Other than client cards what kind of record keeping is needed?*

A Every penny you spend needs to be recorded along with every sale. Record all payroll expenses, retail sales commissions, rent, utilities, and insurance.

Q *19. Do I need to keep my receipts?*

A Keep receipts on every purchase you make including supplies, rent for your station, phone bills, insurance, salon and station maintenance, cleaning, postage, and license renewals.

Q *20. Do I need to keep financial records?*

A Yes, and keeping all records in order can help you at tax time. Today's computer programs make keeping track of your records very simple. A punch of the button can give you the bottom line. There are several companies in the beauty industry that sell systems for the salon. You can also look into customizing a system at your local computer store.

If you don't have access to a computer, hiring a book-keeping company at the beginning of the year can help expedite your taxes at the end of the year. Planning ahead is the key. Compare the cost of hiring a bookkeeping company to the purchase of a small computer, and see which is more cost effective.

Q *21. How do I manage my appointment book?*

A A neat appointment book is the key to minimal mistakes. Whether you use a salon appointment book that stays at the receptionist's desk or carry your own, it is important to understand appointment book etiquette.

Rule #1: Always use pencil.

Rule #2: Draw a line through the times you don't want to take appointments. If you want to start taking appointments at 10 am, draw a line from the first time on the book up to 10 am. If your last appointment is 5 pm, draw a line under 5 pm through the rest of the day. This will clearly define your working schedule.

Rule #3 Schedule a lunch break by writing "lunch" in the time you wish for your break. It defines the fact you are unavailable during that time slot.

Rule #4: Have your appointment book ready for approximately three months ahead. Clients like to plan ahead and you should be prepared. Go through and draw lines through the days you are not working and define your schedule for the days you are. This will eliminate any scheduling conflicts if your book is done well in advance.

Q *22. What are standing appointments?*

A A standing appointment means reserving the same time each week or bi-weekly for a particular client. These appointments should be written in a different colored pencil, so it is easier to remain consistent from week to week.

The standing client never needs to make appointments unless she needs to reschedule her standing for a special reason. The standing appointment is always there.

Q *23. How do I schedule standings?*

A First, identify the standing client. If a client seems to schedule appointments consistently at the same time, you should suggest a standing. Find a convenient time that the client can consistently come in. In a colored pencil, write the client's name in her standing appointment time for the next several months or up to when your book is done. Explain that she never needs to make another appointment with you unless she needs to change one for a special reason.

Q *24. What if a client can't keep her standing appointment?*

A If a client has difficulty keeping her standing appointments, then she is not a standing client. Explain that she needs to schedule her appointments as she goes to and take the pressure off her. If a client cancels twice in a row, or several times in the course of two months, remove her from the standing client list, and suggest that she book her appointment before she leaves each time.

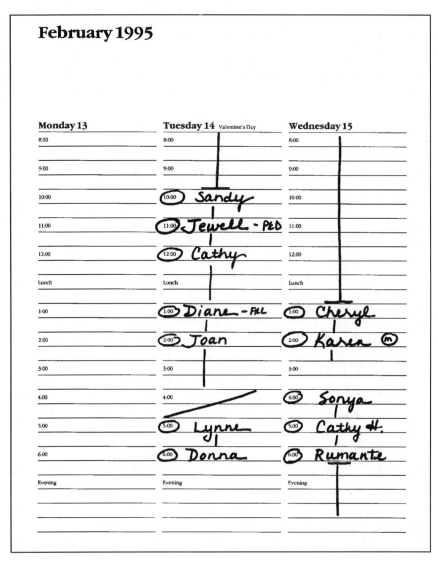

A sample appointment book.

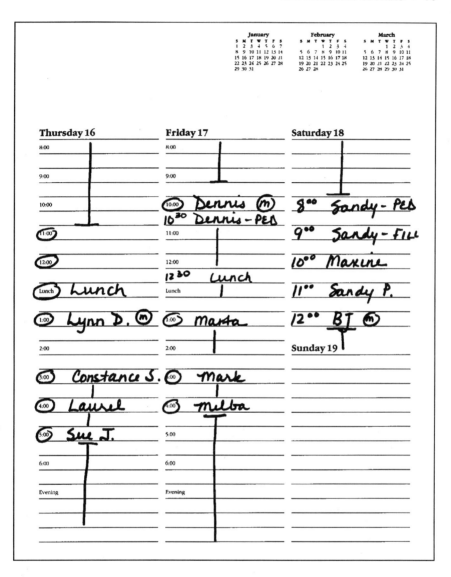

January	February	March
S M T W T F S	S M T W T F S	S M T W T F S
1 2 3 4 5 6 7	1 2 3 4	1 2 3 4
8 9 10 11 12 13 14	5 6 7 8 9 10 11	5 6 7 8 9 10 11
15 16 17 18 19 20 21	12 13 14 15 16 17 18	12 13 14 15 16 17 18
22 23 24 25 26 27 28	19 20 21 22 23 24 25	19 20 21 22 23 24 25
29 30 31	26 27 28	26 27 28 29 30 31

Thursday 16

8:00
9:00
10:00
11:00
12:00
Lunch — Lunch
1:00 — Lynn D. (m)
2:00
3:00 — Constance S.
4:00 — Laurel
5:00 — Sue J.
6:00
Evening

Friday 17

8:00
9:00
10:00 — Dennis (m)
10:30 — Dennis - PED
11:00
12:00
12:30 — Lunch
Lunch
1:00 — Marta
2:00
3:00 — Mark
4:00 — Melba
5:00
6:00
Evening

Saturday 18

8:00 — Sandy - PED
9:00 — Sandy - FILL
10:00 — Maxine
11:00 — Sandy P.
12:00 — BJ (m)

Sunday 19

Promotions

Q 25. *How can I best promote my business?*

A There are many ways of promotion, including advertisements in local newspapers, direct mailings, or by passing out flyers. But the best way of promoting your business is by networking with the existing clientele in the salon. Here are some ideas:

- Give each client several referral cards. They can be business cards with Referred by:_____ written on the back so you know who to thank when the client they referred comes to your salon.
- Send thank you cards to every new client.
- Donate your services to charities and schools.
- Participate in bridal fairs and shows.
- Speak at women groups.
- Participate in Chamber of Commerce activities by donating gift certificates.
- Join a leeds group.
- Network with salons in your area.
- Work promotions at local department stores.
- Offer prom night discounts.
- Donate gift baskets to the Welcome Wagon.
- Provide gifts and special promotional materials to all real estate clients. They are the first person the new neighbor meets.

NOTE: A leeds group is a neighborhood group of business women who meet regularly, often for a breakfast meeting early in the work week. The goal of leeds group members is to network among themselves to generate business.

Retailing

Q *26. Why should I retail?*

A For several reasons. One is to make extra money without working longer hours. Retailing to your clients can increase your income up to 50 percent. Two, you should be offering your clients home nail care so they don't have to purchase their products elsewhere. Three, if your clients use the same products you use, selling retail products can improve the condition of their nails, hands, and feet, making your job easier.

Q *27. What should I retail?*

A Here is a suggested list of items that you can retail focuing on nail and foot care only. Remember, this is only a fraction of what you can retail. Hair care products, skin care, and makeup are easy add ons.

Nail glue
Nail menders such as "Crack Attack"
Cuticle oils
Lotions
Sloughing lotions
Nail brushes
Files
Buffers
Top coats
Base Coats
Quick drying top coats
Polish
Foot care products
Repair kits

Q **28. How do I price the items I retail?**

A Mark each item double what you paid for it. So if you pay $2.00 for a bottle of nail glue, charge at least $4.00.

Q **29. Where do I display the products I will retail?**

A Where the client can see them when they get their nails done. Your client should be able to see the products from her chair at your table. You should also have one weekly special displayed on your desk.

Q **30. Where do I buy the products I retail?**

A Purchase these products from full service distributors that service your areas. Tell the sales person that you would like the best deals and offer to purchase in larger quantities to get the best price. Ask them for upcoming specials so you can plan ahead and stock up when the specials are available.

Another option is to buy at trade shows. You can sometimes find show specials that you will not find at distributor houses. Spend the day at the show shopping around before you buy. If you wait to purchase at the end of the show, the dealer may be willing to bargain if you buy in bulk. The less they have to pack up, the happier most exhibitors are, and they are sometimes willing to sell at lower prices at the end of the show.

Be sure to bring something sturdy in which to carry your products home.

Q **31. Can I get free samples to try before I buy?**

A You can ask. Most manufacturers have sample sizes and most distributors carry them. Sometimes the distributors have to pay for them and if you can't get a free sample ask to pay their price for one.

Q *32. How much money can I make from retailing?*

A If you have a pretty full book, you will probably see any where from 25 to 40 people per week, or an average of 32 clients per week. On a two-week cycle, that is 64 clients total. If you sold each one of them a $4 glue twice a year, that is a net profit of $256 just on glue!

The retail profit is what you make of it. If you sell higher end products that the clients cannot get anywhere else, your retail is doing them a service as well as making you more money. Retail profits can be endless. It is what you make of it.

Q *33. How do I package the products I sell?*

A It is very important that you package your products properly to make the sale credible. Use bags with your salon logo and phone number on it, tags printed with your salon logo, or labels designed for your own private-label products.

Remember that the more you label your products and bags, the more exposure you get.

Q *34. Should I have labels made with my salon name on them for the products I retail?*

A Absolutely. There are several industry affiliated compa-nies that can help you with labels, or you can go directly to a label making company.

Q *35. Should I have bags made with my salon name on them?*

A Yes, a large percentage of the bags are reusable, and that is free advertising for you. You can purchase bags for as little as 25 cents each.

Q *36. Where do I find labels and bags?*

A Consult the nail or beauty industry's trade publications. *NailPro Magazine*'s November issue is their yearly Gold Book and *Nails Magazine* prints an annual Fact Book. Each lists the who's who of the industry and is an index to all products, manufacturers, and distributors related to the nail industry.

Selling Techniques

Q *37. I am not a salesman so how do I sell?*

A Tell, don't sell. Tell the client about the product that is easy and comfortable to use. The product will sell itself if you believe in it and present it right.

Q *38. I am afraid that the client will say no, so what do I do?*

A Don't take it personally. Explain what the product does and why you believe in it. Let her know that if she changes her mind, it is always available.

Q *39. When is the best time to sell?*

A As you are using the product. A description of the product and its benefits is a perfect way to familiarize the client with it. Another good time is when the client asks for a solution to a problem she may be having. Explaining the options she has with the products you sell is a perfect opportunity.

Q 40. *How do I comfortably approach the sale?*

A At the end of the service. Ask if there is anything else she needs. Offer suggestions such as nail glue or cuticle oil. Offer a special if she purchases both. Or you might say, "I have a new cuticle oil I would love for you to try. My other clients have been getting great results from it."

Place the products on your manicuring table so she can see them. Explain the benefits and tell her the price.

Q 41. *How do I close the sale?*

A When she is ready to pay, ask her if you can add them to her bill. Assume the sale. If she does not want the products she will say so, and you can let her know they are there if she should need them.

Q 42. *Should I warranty my work if I sell products to complement my services?*

A Absolutely. It is a hook for the sale and if the client is faithfully using the products, her hands and nails will improve which will make your job easier.

Q 43. *How do I keep track of my sales?*

A If you are not computerized, a duplicate sales slip is necessary: one for the client and one for your records. Generic sales slips can be purchased at office supply stores.

Q 44. *What if another technician sells the product for me?*

A You must establish a percentage payable to the technician. Keep good records and pay commissions weekly or monthly.

Q 45. *How do I keep inventory?*

A If you are computerized, it is simple. Whenever a client purchases an item, it automatically comes out of your inventory when you put the sale in her customer file. Doing inventory is now as simple as pressing a button. If you are doing it manually on paper, it is a bit more time consuming. A quick look in the stock room will let you know what you need. Good record keeping with receipts will also help.

TIP: *In the Bag* by Carol Phillips is a great book to read if you are serious about retailing. This easy-to-read book will help you overcome your fear of selling; see how easy and profitable it can be for you!

Nail Notes

Nail Notes

Extra Education

Professional Organizations

Q *46. What organizations are available for nail technicians to join?*

A American Beauty Association (ABA)
1-800-950-8707
Nail Technicians of America
1-314-534-7980
Nail Industry Association
1-800-326-2457
National Cosmetology Association
1-314-543-7980
National Nail Technician's Group (NNTG)
1-516-266-6684

Q *47. How will joining an organization benefit me and my career?*

A Any industry affiliation can enhance your career by keeping you abreast of what is happening. Fashion trends, statistics, newsletters, educational opportunities, conferences, and trade shows are all items that industry organizations offer.

Q **48. What kind of yearly dues will I be required to pay?**

A They can range anywhere from $1 to $200. Most are pretty reasonable, and they give you plenty of value for your money.

Q **49. What will I get for my money?**

A When joining an organization, the group should define exactly what you will get. A benefits brochure that outlines each and every benefit should be available.

Among the benefits are product discounts, liability insurance, health insurance a lower group rate, continuing education courses, trade publications, admittance to the organization's trade shows, and information about fashion trends.

Q **50. Should I belong to more than one?**

A You should belong to as many as you wish. The more organizations you belong to, the more you can enhance your education and industry affiliation. Each organization has a common goal of serving the industry, but each has its own agenda.

Continuing Education

Q **51. Is there any continuing education available to nail technicians?**

A Yes, all over the world. Many classes are offered through manufacturers, distributors, trade shows, and educational events. In addition, several trade publications and independent educators offer courses.

Q *52. Where do I find such classes?*

A Consult your local distributor for a class schedule. Check with trade shows in your area for brochures that outline the classes they offer. Check trade publications for listings of educational events. Contacting a manufacturer if you're interested in a specific product will lead you to their educator or to a distributor in your area who can also give you a schedule.

Q *53. How do I find accredited classes?*

A There are several organizations and many individual educators who are accredited. However, you must research each one to find out if classes are accredited. Your state board of cosmetology can guide you to these classes. More importantly, they can tell you which classes are required by the state boards to continue your license.

Q *54. How do these accredited classes affect my license?*

A Some states require certain classes and a given amount of hours per year in order to keep your license current. If this is a license requirement, your state board of cosmetology can help you.

Q *55. What is a product-related class?*

A A product-related class is sponsored by a manufacturer and is sales driven. The instruction is on how to use their products only. Usually hosted by a distributor in the area, the class is led by a manufacturer's educator, who instructs the class on the chemical and technical background of the products. Sometimes there is a fee, but other times, for the purchase of a kit, you receive the instruction free.

Q 56. *What is a non product-related class?*

A A non product-related class is technical in nature, and not sponsored by a manufacturer. These classes are harder to come by because they are not sponsored and must be marketed by an independent educator.

Q 57. *Are there benefits to both?*

A Yes, definitely. It is important that we as technicians understand everything we can about the chemicals we work with. That information is best provided by the manufacturer and their educators, who know them best.

In a non product-related class, the focus is on application, the differences among the products, and how to improve your skills. In addition, there should be information about manufacturers and tricks of the trade.

Trade Shows

Q 58. *Where do I find out about trade shows?*

A Ask your local distributors if they know what trade shows will be in your area. Other salons or your colleagues also may know.

Q 59. *What do the trade shows offer?*

A Trade shows are the most important tool in your career. Manufacturers and distributors collectively display and sell their products in an educational forum, usually at a convention center or an exhibit hall at a large hotel. They offer samples, industry information, and new products. You also can see demonstrations and network with some of the leading technicians.

Q 60. *How many are there?*

A It depends on your area. For the most part, you should be near approximately two trade shows a year.

Q 61. *How big are the shows?*

A It depends on the sponsor, and whether it is mainly a nail show or one that has hair and skincare too. A good size nails-only show will have approximately 75 booths and 2,000 attendees over a two-day period.

Q 62. *Who sponsors the shows?*

A That depends. There are really several types of sponsors. A distributor can sponsor a show featuring only the companies that the distributor represents. It is usually closed to other distributors or independent exhibitors and targets only their customers. Sometimes a one-day distributor show can attract up to 1000 attendees for a show with 25 to 30 booths.

The publication *American Salon* produces the International Beauty Show in New York, Dallas, Seattle, and Atlanta. This event is open to all exhibitors and companies, and has over 750 booths. Its intent is to attract attendees from all over the world. Past shows have attracted more than 100,000 people.

The private sponsor who is not representing a manufacturer or distributor can also produce a show. The size of the show depends on the area's demographics and the number of distributors who participate.

Another potential sponsor is a trade organization such as the National Cosmetology Association. Each state has an affiliate that produces a local state-run show. Once or twice a year, they produce a national show. The Midwest Beauty

Show in Chicago is sponsored by the Chicago Cosmetologists Association.

Q 63. How do I get trade show information?

A Once you locate a show you wish to attend, call and request a brochure, and ask to be put on their mailing list for future shows.

Q 64. What kind of education do trade shows offer nail technicians?

A Again, it depends on the show and what its focus is. Most classes and seminars offered at the show are usually manufacturer-sponsored with a few exceptions. Non product-related seminars and classes require more money and are more difficult to offer. Motivational seminars, business workshops, and sales training are some of the educational events you are more likely to see. Some of the larger hair manufacturers sponsor high-profile educators to lead these classes, which are beneficial to all who attend regardless of whether you currently use their products or not. They are banking you will after you attend these classes.

Q 65. Where do I find information on the classes they offer?

A Usually in the show brochure. If the brochures are not descriptive enough, call the show itself and speak to the person who handles education for the show. They should be able to help you.

Q 66. Is the education free with the purchase of a show ticket?

A A lot of the time it is. Sometimes there is an additional charge.

Q **67. Do I need to sign up for the classes I wish to attend?**

A If there is a sign up, yes. It will ensure that you get into a class. If it does not require pre-registration, arrive early. There is usually a 30-minute break between classes, and you can get there early for a good seat.

Q **68. Do I get a certificate for attending the class?**

A Not always, but you should ask. If for some reason they don't give you one, leave a business card and ask the educator to send you one. Another idea is to call the show and ask that they send you one.

When you do receive your certificate, protect them in a plastic page protector in a three ring binder, unless of course, you choose to frame them.

Q **69. How do I prepare for a trade show?**

A • First, do your homework by getting the brochure and reading all the information. Highlight all the classes and booths you want to see, and be aware of the hours.

• If you are traveling to the show, be sure to make your hotel reservations and flight arrangements as soon as you can. Most larger shows run out of hotel rooms several months prior to the show. They also have special rates for trade show goers negotiated by the show management. There should be a special code in the brochure that you can use when making airline and hotel reservations that will identify the lower rates.

• Next, dress in business-like but comfortable clothes. If you plan to spend two or three days on at the show, you will be on your feet most of time. Bring flats and a comfortable carrying bag for your purchases.

- Plan your day. Pick the classes you wish to attend, and make a schedule you can follow. Leave some time for walking the show floor and enjoying refreshments.

- Make a list of all the booths and their numbers that are must sees!

- Pick up as much literature as you can for reading later. Share this literature with colleagues at your salon who couldn't go to the show.

- Ask lots of questions, and spend time watching and listening to the demonstrations. It is amazing what you can learn from watching another tech do a nail even if you don't like the product. Don't miss a thing.

- Watch the nail competitions, and be sure to see the award winning nails. You will be surprised at what you may see that you can take back to the salon.

- If you are staying at a local hotel, drop off your purchases and recharge yourself with a brief rest. You will be that much more alert to finish the show.

Trade Magazines

Q *70. Where do I find out about industry related trade magazines?*

A Sometimes they exhibit at trade shows. You can also get information at your school before you graduate. Sometimes you will receive free magazines that will want you to subscribe.

Q *71. Which ones should I be reading?*

A You should be reading them all. Each magazine has its own focus even though they target the same readers.

Each one has its own style of reporting and usually different educational and technical stories each month.

Q 72. *Are they monthly magazines?*

A Some are monthly, some bimonthly, and some quarterly.

Q 73. *How do I subscribe?*

A You can sign up at the trade shows where the magazines exhibit. Send in a subscriber card from inside any of the magazines or call their 800 number to subscribe over the phone with a credit card. You can also be billed later.

If you choose to be billed later, you are delaying the arrival of your first magazine. Processing a subscription takes six to 12 weeks from the time you subscribe until you are set up on the next mailing cycle.

Q 74. *What is the general cost of a subscription?*

A Anywhere from $20 to $40 a year.

Q 75. *What can be gained from reading a trade magazine?*

A • Technical education
• Product information
• Press releases
• Trade show updates
• Competition winners

- Calendar of events
- Seminar schedules
- Editorials
- Much more!

Check out these magazines for information on:

. . . full service hair salons:
   Modern Salon
   American Salon
   SalonOvations Magazine

. . . salon management:
   Salon Today

. . . nail salons:
   NailPro
   Nails Magazine
   Nail Show
   Mainly Manicuring

. . . skincare:
   Dermascope
   Skin Inc.
   Les Nouvelles Esthetique

Career Development

Q 76. Are there career opportunities available to nail technicians?

A Yes—many. However, you must have an understanding of what is available and how it can work for you. The opportunities are endless because we are in a relatively new industry that is still growing. New companies, new products, new trade shows, and new education are always in demand and so are the available positions.

Q **77. Are these opportunities full time or part time?**

A They can be both. It depends on the company and the position. Most are part time, which enables you to keep your clientele and take classes on the weekends.

Q **78. When would I work?**

A Most part-time educators teach at local distributors on Mondays and work trade shows from Saturday's set up, the show Sunday and Monday, through breakdown after the show on Monday.

Q **79. What would be my responsibilities?**

A Demonstrations, product sales, and working the booth.

Q **80. What kind of compensation does a manufacturer educator make?**

A Most of the compensation is approximately the same from company to company. The going rate is about $100 per day, with set-up commanding a bit less. Depending on the position you have with the company, you may get a percentage of the sales. Hotel rooms, meals, and transportation are paid for by the manufacturer. Most companies ask that you double up in hotel rooms, and usually make your travel arrangements and accommodations for you.

Q **81. How do I go about finding an educator position?**

A Send your resume to the manufacturers you would like to work for. You can find their addresses by looking in the trade magazines' informational books, or call the 800 number on the products or ads you see. Be sure to include all your qualifications before you became a nail tech, and your goals and commitments to bettering the industry with your education. Most important, follow up your resume with a call to the manufacturer. You may prevent it from landing on the wrong desk, wasting valuable time. It will also let the manufacturer know you are serious about pursuing a career with them.

Q *82. Do distributors have educators?*

A Some do and some don't, depending on the focus of the distributors and how committed they are in their division. Most educators are part time and usually train on Sundays and Mondays, and work shows.

One of the strongest assets an educator can offer a manufacturer or distributor is the combination of sales ability and education. The combination is usually rare and is a tremendous asset to the person looking for an educator position. Nail techs want to talk technical to the sales consultant, and if the consultants do not do nails they will not understand the lingo and are therefore limiting themselves as sales consultants.

Q *83. Can I work for more than one manufacturer?*

A Yes, but it depends on the manufacturers and if you are representing direct competitors. A good educator who sets herself up properly with several products that complement each other can do well. However, when it comes to participating in a show, she may have to spread herself thin in order to represent all the products she carries, or just commit to one for the show.

Q *84. What is a resume and why do I need one?*

A A resume is your calling card and first impression. It says who you are, what you want to achieve, and what you have to offer the employer. It should be brief but descriptive. If you are unsure about putting one together, there are many companies that specialize in writing resumes for a small fee. A simple computer program can help you design a beautiful resume. Consult a friend who has a computer if you don't.

Q *85. How do nail competitions benefit my career?*

A In many ways. First, they improve your technique. What you learn in competition can directly improve your salon nails.

Second, they allow you to network with leading technicians you would otherwise not meet. You will expose yourself to a unique and challenging forum that is accessible only to the inner circle of competitors. Also understand that nail competitors are the best of the best and can only be found collectively in a competition. They are independent and travel all over the country, and meet at trade shows.

Third, nail competitions give you tremendous exposure. The manufacturers watch the competitors, what they use, and whether they win. Winning awards on stage, press notices in major magazines, and industry recognition are all benefits of competing. In addition, you may get job offers, educator positions, print work, and endorsements.

Q *86. What other opportunities are there for a technician who would like to pursue a career away from the manicuring table?*

A Article and book writing, trade show work, association leadership, private education, and consultation are all possibilities.

Nail Notes

_____
_____
_____
_____
_____
_____
_____
_____
_____
_____
_____
_____
_____
_____
_____
_____
_____
_____
_____
_____
_____
_____
_____
_____
_____
_____

Nail Notes

Safety & Health

Local & Federal Safety Codes

Q *87. What is the difference between federal and local safety codes?*

A Federal is national and local is city. Each has standards that you must meet in conducting your business.

Q *88. What exactly falls under these codes?*

A Items such as fire codes, and the number of extinguisher locations, sprinkler systems, bathroom facilities, plumbing, wiring, electrical, exit and fire doors, chemical storage, and building permits.

Q *89. What kind of inspections do I need to do before I open my salon?*

A Contact your local officials for a list of codes, rules, and regulations for operating a salon. Use it as a check list to make sure you have covered everything.

Q *90. What kind of licensing will I need to operate a salon?*

A Check with your state board and local officials to find out exactly what you need and how to go about getting the proper license. They should also know how much each license or permit costs.

Salon Safety

Q *91. What can I do to make my salon safer for my clients and my staff?*

A Good ventilation, good lighting, clear aisles and emergency exits, proper storage of chemicals, and a clean environment are all ways of making your salon safer for you, your employees, and clients.

Q *92. Should I allow children in the salon?*

A I know this is a touchy subject but a child without an appointment should have a babysitter. Unattended children are not safe in the salon. There are too many chemicals present for a child to get into.

Parents should realize that holding a child makes it more difficult for the technician. A child leaning on his mom when she is getting her nails polished is going to inhibit the job. Children naturally touch things and a simple touch of your primer brush, and an innocent rubbing of the eyes can put wet primer right into the child's eyes. Remember most clients leave their kids at home for a reason and do not want to put up with someone else's children in the salon. This is their time and they want to relax.

Q *93. How do I implement the rule of "no children allowed" in my salon?*

A Post a sign by the front desk or politely ask if the child has an appointment. If not, say "I am sorry we do not allow children in the salon for insurance reasons unless they have an appointment."

Q 94. How can I improve the air quality in my salon?

A A good ventilation system in any nail salon is important when trying to keep odors to a minimum. Not only will the environment be more attractive, but this will also help combat overexposure to vapors. Understanding how the ventilation system works will help you use it correctly for best results. So, do your homework and read as much as you can about the system before purchasing it.

If you have an air filter system, know the amount of cubic air space it can clean and the cubic size of your salon. Be sure to research the chemicals the system needs because not all systems work with all chemicals.

Ceiling fans and portable fans at your manicuring stations will only serve to re-circulate the vapors, and spread them around for everyone else to breathe. They do not remove the vapors from your salon.

Air conditioning systems will only serve to re-circulate unless they are set up with filters that remove the vapors or exhaust the vapors outside, bringing in fresh air with the intake.

Table fans with a charcoal filtering system that is changed weekly can also assist in removing the vapors. They must be used to remove the fumes when applying acrylic, and can help keep filing dust to a minimum.

The easiest and most effective way to limit the vapors is to use a trash receptacle with a tight cover that keeps the trash sealed. The medical field uses these trash containers, which can cost up to $45.

The biggest contributor to salon vapors is uncovered trash receptacles and open containers. Close all chemical containers immediately after use and throw away the paper table towel as soon as you are finished. This will also help keep the salon smelling fresh. For more technical information on a ventilation system, contact the Lab Safety Supply at (800) 356-2501. Ask for information on the Fume Extractor and a catalog on all safety products.

Q *95. Should I conduct emergency drills with my staff?*

A Yes, this is a good safety procedure. Just as they do on airplanes before flight, you should review the emergency route with your staff. This will help your staff assist the clients and avoid panic.

Q *96. Should I have an alarm system for my salon?*

A That depends on your needs and your insurance company. Your alarm should be hooked up to an alarm company or the police station for maximum results.

Q *97. Should there be a procedure for the last employee and client out at night?*

A Yes, definitely. Never leave by yourself or allow a client to leave the salon at night unescorted. Leave together for safety reasons.

Q *98. How do I safely deposit salon income without risk?*

A First, don't be too consistent about the time you go to the bank. Someone may be aware of your routine. Get someone to go with you and be aware of everyone around you when depositing the money.

First Aid

Q *99. What should a salon or technician have prepared for first aid?*

A A first aid kit should always be filled with the necessary bandages, antiseptics, and emergency items. Include provisions in case of a disaster, such as water, blankets, radio, batteries, flashlights, etc. . . . All Material Safety Data Sheets (MSDS) should be filed in a notebook under category headings.

Q 100. What if the salon owner doesn't have anything prepared?

A Ask that she purchase one. If she is not interested, then you should reevaluate your working environment, the available safety equipment, and the MSDS.

Q 101. Where should the first aid kit be kept?

A It depends on the salon's safety requirements. Common sense suggests the front desk or bathroom.

Q 102. Should there be first aid training in the salon?

A Yes, as in any working environment. Once a year or as part of a new employee's orientation, review the location of the first aid kit, the fire extinguisher, and emergency doors. Emergency procedures and earthquake preparedness also should be reviewed.

Q 103. Where do you learn CPR?

A Contact the local hospital, Red Cross, or fire station for information on classes.

Q 104. What should I do if we have a chemical emergency in the salon?

A Consult the MSDS pertaining to that chemical and follow the instructions.

MSDS

Q *105. What is the MSDS?*

A The MSDS is a Material Safety Data Sheet that accompanies most products.

Q *106. What is the purpose of the MSDS?*

A Federal law requires that manufacturers provide you with important information about a product such as directions for proper use, safety precautions, and a list of active ingredients. Federal regulations require that you be given this information on what is called the Material Safety Data Sheet (MSDS). Each salon is required to have an MSDS for every product that contains a potentially hazardous ingredient.

The Occupational Safety and Health Administration's MSDS format has 40 sections, including but not limited to emergency phone numbers, poison control center, chemical identity, safe exposure limits, harmful by-products, proper storage conditions, health hazards, short and long term effects, signs and symptoms of overexposure, ventilation required, and other precautions for safe use.

Q *107. Who prints the MSDS?*

A It is the manufacturer's responsibility, but guidelines for fulfilling this responsibility are governed by OSHA.

Q *108. Where does the information come from?*

A The manufacturer gathers the information from the company that sells them the products, or from their chemist if the product is made by the manufacturer.

Q *109. If I have a question who do I contact?*

A Call the manufacturer directly. Most nail companies have an 800 number that appears on the container and a staff available for technical questions.

Q *110. Whose responsibility is it to distribute them?*

A It is the responsibility of the organization that sells the product to the person who actually uses the product. For instance, if you purchase a product at a trade show from the manufacturer, the manufacturer should supply the MSDS. If you buy from a supply house, the supply house must furnish the MSDS. If you buy your products from the salon owner, she must supply them. However, you must ask for the MSDS in order to get one. No one is going to assume you want one.

Q *111. What do I do if I cannot get the MSDS on a product I wish to purchase?*

A Call the company directly and ask for one. If your efforts aren't rewarded with an MSDS, maybe you should purchase your products from another company.

Q *112. Do I need one with every purchase?*

A No, as long as the ingredients haven't changed, it is not necessary to get one every time you buy the product.

Q *113. What do I do with them once I have accumulated them?*

A File them in a notebook under sections such as acrylic powders, acrylic monomers, primers, sanitation systems, glue, polish, etc.

Hazardous Materials

Q *114. What are hazardous materials?*

A Everything from liquid monomer to acetone can be considered hazardous. However, when they are used and disposed of properly, they are not hazardous. If you stock 10 gallons of acetone in your back room, you need to understand how to properly store this amount to make the salon safe. Read all your labels, understand what you are working with, and learn how to dispose of the products correctly. There are many products we use regularly in the salon that should not be poured down the drain anymore. If you do not understand the labels, call the manufacturer and ask. There should be a number on the container.

Q *115. How do I take care of chemicals considered hazardous?*

A Each container should be stored in a clean, cool storage area, away from your working station. Containers should not be clear, thus protecting the chemical from the environment which can weaken their strength. Each bottle should be labeled with the date of purchase for proper rotation. You should also be aware if there is an expiration date.

Q *116. What about storing these chemicals?*

A Ask your manufacturer or distributor for an MSDS which should give you the proper storage procedures. You may also contact your local fire department and ask procedures you need to take for safe storage. Ask them to come and inspect your salon frequently. They will be more than willing to help.

Q *117. How do I dispose of the hazardous chemicals?*

A Do not pour nail liquid (monomer) or used acetone down the sink drains or toilets in your salon. There are chemical disposal companies that do nothing but dispose of used acetone and other products you are using. Call them and have them pick up your hazardous waste properly. It will be safer for everyone.

The best way to dispose of acrylic liquid is to mix 1 part powder to 1 part liquid and let the product dry in small balls on your table towel. Then you can throw them away safely. Do this in small amounts only since large amounts can be unsafe. Avoid waste by pouring only as much liquid as you need.

Q *118. Does the fire department monitor hazardous chemicals?*

A Yes they do. They also carry out random salon inspections that you need to be prepared for. Contact your local fire department and state board for requirements on the storage of chemicals such as acetone. Also consider giving a floor plan to the fire department identifying chemical and hazardous waste storage areas.

Q *119. What do I do if I think I have a problem with some hazardous material?*

A Consult your MSDS, the manufacturer, or the poison control unit in your area.

Nail Notes

Nail Notes

Bacteria/Infectious Diseases

AIDS Awareness

Q *120. The big question is, can I really get AIDS from doing nails?*

A It is not likely. If you practice good sanitation procedures in the salon at all times and understand exactly what you are dealing with you can educate yourself as to when you are at risk.

Q *121. How do I protect myself and my clients from any risk?*

A Good sanitation and disinfection practices and common sense.

Q *122. What should I tell my clients when they ask if they can catch AIDS?*

A Tell them they have nothing to fear because you practice good sanitation with each and every client. Explain that no one catches AIDS, but rather the HIV virus. HIV is a fragile virus that is difficult to spread. It can be spread through blood contact on an open sore, wound, or mucous membranes, but not by just touching the blood. They can become HIV positive only in the worst case scenario. Educate yourself on how HIV is transmitted and then teach your clients. The fear is the unknown; put your clients at ease with your knowledge.

Q 123. Where do I get the truth about how to catch HIV?

A Read *HIV/AIDS & Hepatitis* by Douglas Schoon. This book was written specifically for the salon industry.

Q 124. Can I safely manicure an HIV client?

A Yes, you can. Do not cut cuticles and make them bleed, and be sure to use good sanitation practices. However, you may never know if your client is HIV positive or not, so you should always be careful.

Q 125. Can I really transmit diseases on my metal implements?

A Yes. It is difficult, but possible.

Q 126. Can I transmit diseases on my files?

A Bacteria and fungal spores are everywhere. A high concentration of these spores or bacteria is what causes disease. If you are filing into a colony of these spores or bacteria (for example, a spot on the cuticle that looks infected or inflamed) you can transplant the colony, spreading the infection.

Files cannot support life, but depending on the type of bacteria or spores and how long they live, it is possible, though unlikely, to transmit these germs.

Q *127. Should I take extra precautions with the file I use?*

A Yes. Working in a clean environment and using sanitized or new files for each client will help prevent any spread of bacteria or spores. Do not work on a client who has red or swollen cuticles, or an open cut. If you happen to cut the client when filing be sure to throw the file away after you finish. Do not use the file on another client.

Hepatitis

Q *128. How does one catch Hepatitis?*

A There are several types of hepatitis and each is transmitted differently, mostly by blood, sex, or sharing needles.

Q *129. What are the symptoms?*

A Hepatitis affects the liver of an infected person. The first symptoms of hepatitis infection are typically fever, nausea, stomach pain, loss of appetite, aching, and constant fatigue. Sometimes the urine turns brown. Often, the white parts of the eyes become yellow. The skin may also appear yellow. The symptoms of an infected liver are tenderness and swelling of the liver.

Q *130. How do you identify the client who has hepatitis?*

A You don't. But if the client tells you she has hepatitis, don't panic. Taking all the routine precautions will protect you both. However, if you are not practicing good sanitation procedures, you are putting yourself and the rest of your clients at risk.

Q *131. What precautions do I need to take in order to protect myself?*

A Practicing good sanitation procedures is the best protection of all.

Q *132. Can I safely manicure a client with hepatitis?*

A Yes, but you should avoid cutting any cuticles. Do not manicure any client who has open cuts. Use common sense when manicuring anyone who may present a risk.

Viruses & Colds

Q *133. How do I protect myself form catching the common cold and viruses in the salon?*

A You can protect yourself simply by staying healthy. The most important protection is to always wash your hands between clients. Washing drastically reduces the chances of catching a cold or virus. Insist that your clients wash their hands upon arrival, and if they have a cold, not to cough into their hands while you're working on them. Give them tissues instead.

Q *134. When do I refuse to work on a client who has a cold?*

A When the client is visibly sick. Use your common sense when making this decision and reschedule the appointment. Remember that everyone in the salon is exposed when a sick client comes to your salon.

Q **135. How do I refuse the client because she is sick?**

A Diplomatically of course. Ask her to reschedule. Explain that you are concerned for other clients and techs in the salon.

Q **136. If I am sick, should I not work?**

A If you have a cold, you should not work at all.

Q **137. Should I wear a mask?**

A If you feel it's necessary, wear a mask. Dab the inside of the mask with some Vicks Vapor Rub to help clear your breathing. Wear a new mask for 1 day and then throw it away. Again, good sanitation practices and common sense can keep you from catching colds and viruses in the salon.

Q **138. Should my sick client wear a mask?**

A Yes, if you feel it's necessary. Ask your client diplomatically and explain that it will benefit you and your other clients. You may want to wear one with her to make her feel more comfortable. Throw away the masks after the appointment.

Q **139. Do gloves protect me from getting a cold from a client?**

A They can assist in protecting you but washing your hands is more effective. Be sure to change gloves for each new client.

Q 140. What other viruses am I susceptible to in the salon?

A There are many viruses that we are susceptible to both in and out of the salon. The key is to practice good sanitation procedures at all times, which is the best protection of all. Work reasonable hours. If you have a healthy lifestyle you will be taking the right steps to ensure your safety.

Mold & Fungus

Q 141. Are fungus and mold contagious?

A Yes, both are contagious. They can spread from nail to nail on the client, and from the client to the nail technician.

Q 142. What is a mold?

A Mold is a fungus infection of the nail that is usually caused when moisture seeps between an artificial nail and the free edge of the nail.

Q 143. What does mold look like?

A Usually a thriving fungus infection has medium green color. A more vibrant green/turquoise color means it is getting worse; the next stage would be black.

Q 144. What causes the fungus infection?

A Everyday moisture from exposure to water, which can come from washing your hands, doing dishes, or taking showers. Water gets trapped between the natural nail and the lifted acrylic, creating a warm dark place for the fungus to breed.

Q 145. *How do I cure it?*

A Curing is killing. Remove by lifting or soaking the artificial product off the affected nail. In a more severe case, remove the product entirely. Gently buff the natural nail with a soft or fine file and remove as much discoloration as possible without damaging the natural nail.

The exposure to air is enough to kill the bacterial infection. The reason it grows underneath the artificial product is that its air is cut off and it can thrive in a warm dark place. As soon as you expose it to the air, it dies.

The discoloration is a stain that may not come out completely, depending on the age of the bacterial infection. It will have to grow out. Throw away the file you used, and sanitize all implements. Clean the nail with a nylon brush and an antibacterial soap. Dry the nails thoroughly and apply a dehydrant before applying primer and reapplying the product. The use of acetone is not necessary. Soaking the nail in bleach is not recommended and is hazardous to the skin. Iodine, over-the-counter fungus products, and hydrogen peroxide are also not necessary and will serve only to help keep the nails clean.

Q 146. *How do I prevent mold and fungus infection from happening?*

A Perfect your application technique to the point that you have no lifting at all. This may sound impossible but it is not. Time and practice will play a big part on product retention as well as finding the right product that works well for you.

Minimizing lifting is the goal. Having your client maintain her nails on a regular basis will help. Preparing the nail for acrylic applications, and using dehydrants and preventatives also can help.

Q 147. *What is a fungus?*

A Fungi is the general term for vegetable parasites including all types of fungus and mold.

Q 148. *What causes fungus?*

A Trauma, abuse from removing nails too often, medications, allergies, and several other reasons can be the cause of fungi. Some are curable and some are not, some are permanent and some temporary.

Q 149. *What does fungus look like?*

A It usually appears as a discoloration in the nail that spreads toward the cuticle. As the condition matures, the discoloration becomes darker.

Q 150. *Can I treat a fungus?*

A No, it goes beyond our manicuring license, and you must refer the client to a doctor, dermatologist, or podiatrist. But don't let them tell your client that acrylic nails are bad. They are fine if done correctly. Invite the doctor for a complimentary manicure, and educate him on your services.

Knowing where your manicurist license ends and a doctor's begins is where you should draw the line. We are not licensed to diagnose, so we should know when to work on the nail and when not to. Milady's book *The Art and Science of Nail Technology* explains it best with the "Golden Rule." The "Golden Rule" is, that if the nail or skin to be worked on is infected, inflamed, broken, or swollen, a nail technician should not service the client. Instead refer the client to a doctor. Build a relationship with your local doctors for referrals and work with them. Your insurance should cover any liability problems that occur.

Q *151. How do I prevent fungus?*

A You don't, but there are some precautionary measures you can take. Proper sanitation procedures should always be practiced at your manicuring table. When removing artificial products, cause as little trauma to the natural nails as possible. Proper nail preparation and scrubbing is the most important precaution.

Q *152. What can I do to educate clients?*

A Assure them they are in a safe environment, and explain how you clean your implements, sanitize your station, and care for their safety.

Tell your clients what they can expect from your nail care, and how you handle problems should they arise. Educate them on the importance of regular maintenance. Tell them they can feel free to see you when they have broken a nail. Talk about the products you use, why you like them, and how they benefit their nail services.

Fear is not knowing. If you have an educated client, she will not worry about your nail services.

Nail Disorders

Q *153. What exactly is a nail disorder?*

A It is a disturbance of the natural growth pattern that usually causes structural damage.

Q **154. What are the specific terms of common disorders?**

A **Onychosis** is any disease or deformity of the nail.

Onychia is nail bed inflammation.

Paronychia is inflammation of the cuticle and tissue surrounding the nail bed.

Periungual is the tissue or area around the nail plate.

Subungual is the tissue or area under the nail plate.

Q **155. What are some of the more common nail disorders?**

A **Beau Lines** (Transverse Lines)—Depressions extending from one side of the nail to the other. True beau lines usually affect all the nails and are caused by systemic diseases. They are the result of the temporary cessation of nail growth. Injury can cause a similar condition but usually only the injured nail is affected.

Blue Nails—The nail plate may appear blue because of the lack of oxygen to the subungual tissues. Some drugs may cause the nail plate to appear blue or blue-gray in color.

Bruised Nails—Trauma or injury to the nail results in a dark blue or black color under the nail plate. The color is due to bleeding under the nail. A fresh injury is red or dark bluish in color, and as the blood clots, it turns black.

Eggshell Nails—These have the appearance of an egg shell. They are thin, fragile, and whitish in color. They curve over the free edge. The cause may be improper diet, medications, disease, or even acute psychotic disorders.

Spoon Nails (Koilonychia)—The edges of these nails turn up making the central portion of the nail a concavity or "spoon" shaped. The most common causes of this nail disorder are occupational contact with oils and other distillates and chemicals, and iron deficiency.

Leukonychia (white nail)—A whitish discoloration of the nail plate. May be classified as either true or apparent. True leukonychia is the actual discoloration of the nail plate. This can be caused by congenital factors such as minor injuries to the nail bed. The most common form seen is the small white spots in the nail plate due to repeated minor injuries to the nail bed. Apparent leukonychia is where the nail plate does not adhere to the bed because of injury or diseases like fungal infections under the nail. The loose portion of the nail appears white because light is refracted differently through it.

Onychatrophy—A reduction of the normal size of the nail plate often associated with fragmentation and splitting of the nail. The nail begins as a normal nail and reduces in size because of chronic nail biting or psoriasis of the nail. Even severe cases of paronychia can cause a reduction of size.

Onychogrytosis—A thickening of the nail plate. The most apparent form is "Rams Horn" nail which results from injuries. Other causes are congenital, infections, poor circulation, and long-term repeated minor injuries from improperly fitted shoes.

Oncholysis—Detachment of the nail plate from its underlying bed. Common causes are injuries, and fungal or bacterial infections of the nail bed.

Onychomycosis—A fungal infection of the nail apparatus which can include the nail plate, nail bed, and the tissues surrounding the nail, alone or in any combination. The fungal infection may cause nail disorders such as onychogryphosis, onycholysis, leukonychia, etc.

Onychorrhexis—A series of narrow parallel grooves extending from the base of the nail plate to its free edge. Splitting is common in the grooves. Seen in diseases of the nail such as lichen planus and psoriasis. Also caused by occupational trauma.

Onychia—An inflammation of the nail bed, resulting in the loss of the nail.

Paronychia—An inflammation or infection involving the folds of tissue surrounding the nail, usually caused by bacteria or fungi.

Platonychia (Pincer or Trumpet Nail)—Defined as an over curvature of the nail margins. The greatest curvature is noted at the free edge of the nail margin and may be so great that the underlying nail bed is entrapped in the curve of the nail, thus the term Trumpet Nail. Causes may be old age, neglect, injury, etc.

Splinter Hemorrhage—Small (2–3mm long) deposits of blood seen under the nail plate. When first formed they are reddish in color (fresh blood) but within two to three days, turn black as the blood coagulates. They then look like a small splinter under the long axis of the nail plate. Minor injury is the most common cause. If multiple splinter hemorrhages are seen in several nails, the cause may be bacterial endocarditis (an infection of the heart).

Onyccgocryptosis (Ingrown nail)—The margin of the nail curves into the nail groove. The nail then penetrates the skin resulting in an infection (paronychia, onychia). Causes are congenital malformation of the nail bed, injuries, improperly fit shoes, and inadequate trimming of the nail.

Q *156. How do I handle a client who has a nail disorder?*

A Assess the problem first so you know exactly what is wrong and whether it's an infection or physical problem. You do not want to hurt the client or work on infected nails.

Q *157. Can I safely manicure or apply artificial products to a client who has a nail disorder?*

A If the problem is physical and not infected, you can safely apply products and manicure them. Eczema is a good example. If the client's nail beds are rough and bumpy, you can apply acrylic safely over the roughness and give the client a smoother nail.

Q *158. When should I not manicure a client with a disorder?*

A When the nails are obviously sore and red, with puss, swelling, a fungal infection, or lifting off the nail plate.

Q *159. Is there any home care treatment that I can recommend to the client?*

A We are not doctors and you should leave this up to the dermatologist. But you should suggest she file the problem nails to keep them short.

Nail Notes

Nail Notes

Infection Control

Chemical Sanitation

Q 160. What is sanitation?

A It is the minimal form of disinfection and the reduction of pathogenic organisms with a disinfectant soap and water solution.

Q 161. What should I be using in the salon to sanitize my implements?

A A liquid solution that will sanitize your implements by submersion, thereby sanitizing your work area and salon.

Q 162. Should I be doing more than just sanitizing?

A Yes, it is important that you wash your implements before submerging them in the solution. You must remove all skin tissue and debris, otherwise all you are doing is contaminating the solution.

Q 163. What is disinfection?

A Disinfection means killing all disease-causing organisms on your work surfaces and implements.

Q *164. What is sterilization?*

A It is the elimination of all spores and bacteria, leaving nothing alive. This is the highest level of disinfection and not necessary for the salon.

Q *165. What is the biggest misconception in salon sanitation?*

A Not understanding the exact usage of the disinfection solution and its purpose. Understand that all solutions are not created equal, and each may have its own directions for usage. Learn the strengths and usage of the different solutions. The labels will state what it kills.

Q *166. What is the most important thing to remember when sanitizing?*

A Follow the procedures precisely and be faithful to them. Sanitize between each client. Use a clean implement to retrieve the ones in the solution. Change the solution when it gets cloudy or when time permits. Wash the implements prior to sanitizing.

Q *167. How do I know I have a strong enough product?*

A Read the labels for what the solution kills and follow the instructions.

Q *168. Where do I get the proper guidelines on what to use?*

A Your state board can provide them. If you choose to take extra measures, research the products and read up on this issue.

Q *169. Where do I purchase the solution I need for the salon?*

A You can get it from your local distributor or directly from the manufacturer.

Physical Sanitation

Q *170. What do I need to do physically to ensure I am working within sanitary guidelines?*

A
- Start with good table practices. Have you and your clients get in the routine of washing hands thoroughly before each service. You, the technician, need to wash your hands between each client also.
- Don't take the client's excuse that she washed her hands before she came. That is not good enough anymore. She turned the doorknob her kids touch with their dirty hands everyday and as she left, she got out her dirty keys. She touched the steering wheel, which is not necessarily clean and read the newspaper while she waited for you. Her hands may appear to be clean but they are not.
- Don't be intimidated by asking her to wash her hands. Ease the situation by washing your hands along with her, and explain that it protects both of you. She will appreciate it and get right into the routine.
- Always use clean implements that have not been used on another client.
- Do not allow your client to put her hands to her face, rub her eyes, cover her mouth to cough, etc. without washing her hands again. That goes for you too.

PART TWO

The
Technical
Side

Natural Nails

The Manicure

Q 171. What are the basic steps for the manicure?

A First, have your clients wash their hands and exfoliate them before they sit down. Prepare your manicure soak with warm soap and water and always have clean table towels available.

Step 1 Remove nail polish on all 10 nails.

Step 2 File and shape all the nails on the left hand, then soak it while you file the right hand.

Step 3 Take the left hand out of the water and soak the right hand.

Step 4 Apply cuticle cream to the left hand. Gently push the cuticles back and trim what is necessary.

Step 5 Remove the right hand from the water. Apply cuticle cream and push cuticles back and trim if necessary.

Step 6 Massage the hands and arms to the elbow.

Step 7 Clean the nail plate and under the nails with soap and water.

Step 8 Remove any lacy edges and trim anything else that needs trimming.

Step 9 Polish 1 base coat, 2 coats of color and a top coat.

Q *172. What is the best maintenance for natural nails?*

A Essentially, a basic manicure is the best way to keep natural nails healthy, growing, and in good shape. There is no magic in a bottle that can replace the benefits of a manicure on a regular basis.

Q *173. How often should nails be manicured?*

A For maximum results, manicure nails weekly. Every other week can be effective, but a weekly manicure will give the best results.

Q *174. Are there any products that can be applied to make the nails harder and to make them grow?*

A No, absolutely not, but they can all help. The magic is in the manicure itself combined with a good base and top coat.

Q *175. What are the best products to use on natural nails?*

A Natural nail care systems developed by manufacturers that are specifically for natural nails. There are several companies that have very good base and top coats, cuticle creams, and hand lotions that work in conjunction with each other to provide you a good system to use for maximum results.

Q *176. Is there anything special I should do when performing a manicure?*

A Yes, there is. Use a hot oil manicure if your client has dry hands and nails. Take care in trimming the nails and pushing the cuticles back. Be gentle and rub the cuticles every time you apply an oil or lotion to stimulate their growth. The massage is very important so don't shortchange the client on this.

Other than the basics, the important thing to remember is the detail work on every step you take. A manicure should "clean up and maintain" the nails, so there should not be a hang nail or a rough edge when done.

Q *177. Is there anything else I can do for add-on services?*

A Yes. You can add a paraffin wax before the manicure, a hand facial with glycolic acid lotions, reflexology, or a wax for the hair on the fingers. Those are just some suggestions and ways to add on to the basic manicure.

Q *178. What are some of the extra steps I can take in performing a good manicure?*

A • First and foremost, all your tools should be clean, fresh from your sanitizer. Let the client see that you have cleaned them before use.

- Use a soft clean file when filing the nails. Too many times we see coarse acrylic files used for a natural nail manicure. Your grit should be a 240 or higher, depending on the nails. Here is where you should take extra care using clean files.

- Use a soft fine pumice or hindu stone to go over the edges for a smoother finish. This will give the nails a finished quality that you cannot get from the file, and remove the lacy edges that sometimes elude us. A pumice or hindu stone used for manicuring or pedicuring is made from the same material, varying in coarseness. Either can be sanitized along with your implements and should be sanitized after every use.

• With a soft buffer or the black side of a three-way buffer, gently buff the natural nail plate. This has two purposes: one, it evens out any ridges that may be on the nails; and two, it gives the polish a better surface to adhere to and helps the polish last longer. However, if you see a client weekly, you need to buff her nails only once a month. If you buff them too often you will only weaken them.

Q 179. Do I need to cut the cuticles?

A No. Do so only if necessary. It is not a requirement to cut cuticles during a manicure. If you soften cuticles, push them back and keep them in good condition, it is not necessary to ever cut them.

Q 180. Can I high-shine the natural nails safely?

A Yes you can. Use a small amount of cuticle oil and buffing cream to enhance the shine. Be sure not to buff too much and too quickly. Buff in one direction only. Buffing quickly heats the nails and will make the client uncomfortable.

Q 181. What is the best home maintenance for a natural nail client to help her polish stay on longer?

A Once you find a top coat that works well in the salon, have your client purchase a bottle for home care. Have her apply 1 thin top coat every night for the first three days after the manicure and then every other day until she feels the need to remove the polish or comes in for another manicure. The key is to head off the chipping with extra coats—not wait until the polish starts chipping. Another way to keep polish looking fresh is to apply the top coat over the edge of the tip where it wears off first from everyday use. Applying a top coat to the tips of the nails, will help prevent the colored polish from wearing off.

The Pedicure

Q *182. What are some of the basic steps of a pedicure?*

A First, prepare the foot bath with a conditioning soap, antiseptic, and warm water, while your client chooses her polish. Make sure your client is comfortable while you are preparing everything.

One of the most important items on your list of tools is a sanitary or new file for each client. Use only sanitized implements and a clean foot bath. None of these things should be overlooked.

Step 1 Soak the feet for approximately 5 to 7 minutes to soften skin and cuticles. Alternate each foot in and out of the foot bath with every procedure, having the client continue to soak between each procedure.

Step 2 Take one foot at a time, remove the polish, and file the nails.

Step 3 Apply cuticle cream. Push the cuticles back and trim if necessary.

Step 4 Buff the top of the natural nails with a gentle buffer to remove any ridges in the toe nails.

Step 5 Remove any callous or dead skin on the bottom of the feet.

Step 6 Exfoliate the feet by using a fine pumice. Remove the pumice from its container with an orangewood stick or spatula. Place it in the palms of your hands and gently rub over the entire foot, removing the dead skin. Rinse the feet to remove the remainder of the pumice before the next step.

Step 7 Massage the feet and legs to the knees.

TIP: Do not have client put feet back in the foot bath.

Step 8 Clean off the nails with soap and water to remove the cuticle lotion and oils. Put in the toe separators.

Step 9 Polish.

Q *183. Can I use the credo blade or razor on her feet?*

A Consult your state board and follow their guidelines pertaining to this technique. If your state board allows the use of a credo or razor, start by practicing on yourself. Always use a new blade for each client and disinfect the tool before each use. Remember, it is better to take off too little than too much.

You can train with another technician on the proper use of the credo blade first. Practicing on yourself will give you a respect for the blade and a firsthand understanding of how much you can cut. Cutting too much can also cause discomfort, so it is better to cut less and finish with a pumice stone or foot file.

Q *184. How do I handle the client who insists on the use of a credo when it is against state board regulations?*

A Explain to the client that you are putting your license and salon at risk by not following state regulations. Assure her that you can perform a good pedicure without one.

Q *185. What if the client has thick hard toenails?*

A You can file or buff them to a better shape as long as it is not uncomfortable to the client.

Q 186. *How do I handle ingrown toenails?*

A Gently press the area around the nail to identify the specific area that is affected. If the nail is extremely sore and infected, you should refer her to a podiatrist. A regular pedicure can help prevent ingrown nails by keeping the nails short and manicured.

First, file the ingrown nail flat across the top of the free edge. You can relieve the pressure on the skin by clipping the curling edges of the nail in the nail grooves by using your nippers. Using a smooth file, finish the edges of the nail you just clipped. With an orangewood stick clean under the nail and along the nail grooves. Remember, the longer the client soaks her foot, the softer the skin, making this procedure more comfortable for the client.

If the client doesn't mind the cosmetic look of cutting a small "V" in the center of the free edge of the ingrown nail, it too will relieve some pressure. Another way to relieve the pressure of an ingrown toe nail is to place a small amount of cotton under the edges of the ingrown nail. This will keep the corners elevated and away from the nail groove.

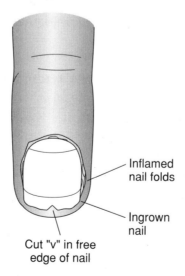

Inflamed
nail folds

Ingrown
nail

Cut "v" in free
edge of nail

To relieve the pressure of an ingrown toenail, cut a small "V" in the center of the free edge.

Q 187. *How long should toenails be?*

A Cosmetically, they should always be short and neat. But first ask the client what shape she prefers, especially on her big toes. The proper shape should be barely a free edge that takes the shape of the toe nail itself. So if the nail bed has an oval look to it file it oval. If the edge for the toe is flat, file it square. Leave a slight free edge if necessary.

Q 188. *When should I refuse to perform a pedicure?*

A When the client's feet aren't sanitary or they have a condition such as athlete's foot or open sores.

Q 189. *How do you identify athlete's foot?*

A Athlete's foot, which is extremely common, can be identified as a fungal infection surrounding the toes and soles of the feet. An itchy dry cracked appearance or blisters are symptoms of athlete's foot. A pedicure should not be performed on a client with athlete's foot because of the high risk of transmission to other clients.

Q 190. *If a client has a corn on her toe what should I do?*

A Corns are beyond our manicuring license and we can not treat them. However, gently, with a soft file, you can smooth the top surface to make the client more comfortable. Over-the-counter medications and donut patches that assist in curing the problems can be used. Consult your local drug store pharmacists for their recommendations on products.

Nail Notes

Nail Notes

Primers

Primers & Their Functions

Q *191. What is a nail primer?*

A It is a chemical product that is applied to the nail plate to enhance the retention of the acrylic product.

Q *192. What is the function of a nail primer?*

A To provide bonding between the acrylic product and the natural nail plate.

Q *193. Do you have to use a nail primer?*

A No, but it is recommended. Some clients can handle a product application to their natural nails without lifting and some can't. For the client whose nails never lift you may be able to skip the primer but it is recommended for the average client whose nails will lift after a few weeks.

Q *194. How is primer applied?*

A Hold the nails at a downward angle. Dip the brush into the primer. Gently touch the brush to your table towel so it can absorb any excess and give you a clear understanding of how much primer is left in your brush. You do not want the extra product to run into the cuticles because it will burn the skin. Gently, with the primer brush on the center of the nail plate well below the cuticle, let a drop flow across the nail plate and wipe the brush to cover any dry areas. The key is to apply sparingly.

Q *195. How many coats of primer are needed to maximize its effectiveness?*

A Two is the maximum needed for good retention, one in the case of the average non-lifter.

Q *196. Can you over prime the nails?*

A Yes, two coats give you maximum results, any more will flood and not improve results.

Q *197. Does the primer burn?*

A Yes, when it touches the skin. It is the cause of most cuticle burning, and the nails should not be touched after the primer is applied by you or the client. If you get it on your finger, it too will burn.

Q *198. How does one get the primer to stop burning?*

A I am not sure there is a way to neutralize it. However I have heard that washing the nail with soap and water or with baking soda helps. I usually apply acrylic to that nail first and massage a conditioning oil on the cuticle to make the client feel more comfortable.

How Primers Work

Q *199. How does an acid primer work?*

A Primers are a form of acid, some slow acting, some fast acting, which is why they burn when they touch the skin. When applied, the primers pit the natural nail, creating pockets in the nail plate for the acrylic to hold on to.

Q *200. How does a non-acid primer work?*

A This kind of a primer is applied like the traditional acid primer and works like the "two-sided sticky tape" method. It sticks to the nail and the acrylic sticks to it.

Q *201. Should I work with the primer wet or dry?*

A You should always follow the manufacturer's directions for the maximum results. I have seen success with both techniques.

Q *202. What products work with primer?*

A All acrylic products and gels can be used with primers for maximum retention.

Q *203. Are there any products that I should not use primer on?*

A Yes, fiberglass does not need a primer and will lift with the use of primer.

Nail Notes

Nail Notes

_____
_____
_____
_____
_____
_____
_____
_____
_____
_____
_____
_____
_____
_____
_____
_____
_____
_____
_____
_____
_____
_____
_____
_____
_____
_____
_____
_____
_____

Filing & Shaping Techniques

Nail Shapes

Q *204. What are the most popular shapes?*

A There are several variations.

Square Is an extremely square tip with straight sides and sharp corners.

Square with Soft Corners Square as in above with straight sides, square tip but soft, barely rounded corners.

Squoval (Square Oval) Straight sides, oval, slightly bowed tip, with soft corners, giving the nail an oval top with straight base.

Oval/Round 50% of the side extending from the stress area is straight out from the nail groove with a slight, tapered graduation with an oval top.

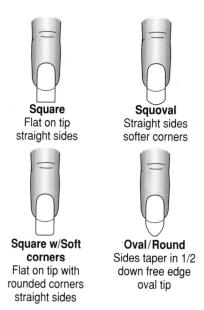

Nail shapes.

Q 205. What is the arch?

A The arch is the graduation of the high point of the nail, which lends strength to the stress area. Viewing the nail from the side, the high point should be located over the natural smile line as the nail leaves the nail bed and becomes the free edge. This is the weakest point of the nail structure, needing the most reinforcement. The arch is the natural shape of the high point of the nail providing the strength over the free edge.

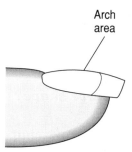

The arch is the high point from the side view.

Q 206. What is the stress area?

A The stress area is where the nail bed and the free edge come together at the natural smile line. The stress area of the nail is where it is the weakest.

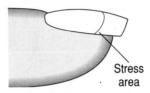

The stress area is where the nail leaves the nail plate and becomes the free edge.

Q 207. What is the sidewall?

A A sidewall is the side of the nail as it extends out from the nail groove.

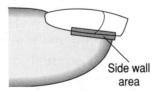

A sidewall is the side of the nail extending out from the nail groove.

Q 208. What is a c-curve shape?

A It is the convex and concave shape of the tip as you look down the barrel of the nail.

Shaping

Q 209. How do I achieve the right shape for each client?

A You must assess the shape of the natural nail bed and fingers before you decide which shape is best for a client. If they are short and fat, you should shape the nails oval with a medium length. If the client has long slender nail beds, they can be longer and square or squoval. Remember, the nails should be an extension of the fingers and the shape should complement the hands. It is easier to build the nails square and try different shapes until you find the best shape for that client.

Q 210. Is there a system to shaping?

A Yes, and it is yours to devise, as long as you are consistent. Here is an example of my system: With a 100 grit file I shape one nail at a time. I shape the parameter first by shaping the left side then the right side, and then the tip. I file the entire top of the nail and then fine tune the cuticle. Then I move on to the next nail and file with the same system. After I file all 10 nails I go over each one with a 180 or softer file before I buff them. This way I get a second look, file things I have missed, and stay with a structured system, which in the long run saves time.

Q 211. What files should I use?

A Start with a coarse, 100 grit file, graduate to a 180 then move on to a 240 or 280 file or block to smooth the nails.

Q 212. How do I get my filing and shaping smooth?

A If you graduate the coarseness properly, you can get a nice finish. If you go from a 100 grit to a white block (approximately 280 grit), you will only soften the finish on the surface of the nail, never buffing out the deep scratches the 100 grit file made. You must graduate your grits in small amounts such as: 100 to 180 to 240 or 280 to a white block. If you go from a 100 to a 240 you will never get a high shine.

Q *213. Should I measure my nails?*

A Always. Keep the index, ring and middle nails approximately the same length. Measure ring to ring, middle to middle and index to index. The thumbs and pinkies should be the same length as each other but in proportion to the others.

Q *214. Should I measure the nails from the underside or the top side?*

A Always topside from the cuticle to the tip. Not all nail beds are created equal and you cannot depend on them to be exactly even.

Q *215. How do I get my nails a consistent shape?*

A With practice and a consistent filing system. If you are all over the place when filing, the nails will have an "all over the place" inconsistent look.

Q *216. Is there a way of checking my filing?*

A Yes, here are five basic guidelines for you to follow.

Top View

Check the overall consistency so the nails match.
Check the shape of the tips.
Measure the nails for consistent length.

Both Side Views

Look for straight edges from all nail grooves on all sides.
Are the sides even?
Do the sides have a finished quality about them?
Is the arch consistently located over the stress area?
Is the high point too close to the cuticle?
Is the tip too heavy?

Down the Barrel of the Nail

Look at the quality of the c-curve.
Is the concave or convex even?
Is the tip too thick or too thin?
Did the form fit tightly under the free edge?
Is the tip on straight?
Is there glue residue underneath?

From the Client's Perspective Turn the client's hand around and view the top of the nail from her perspective and look for flat spots, dips and bumps you can't see from your perspective.

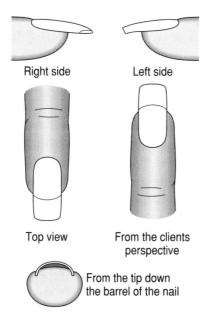

Right side   Left side

Top view   From the clients perspective

From the tip down the barrel of the nail

Five views when checking filing.

BUFFING

Q *217. What files do I need to buff the nails?*

A You should use a black block, a white block, and a three-way buffer file or block, and cuticle oil.

Q *218. If I use a black block buffer, can I get a high shine?*

A First, you should note the coarseness and ask yourself if it is coarser than the last file you used. The black block can come in different coarseness and you need to use a medium side with some cuticle oil to start with. Then graduate your coarseness with a fine side, and then a white block.

Q *219. When I use oil with my white block buffer it ruins it. What do I do?*

A Oils will ruin the white block because it is made of material that the grit is blown on and is more fragile than a traditional black block. Use the oil with a black block, and wipe the excess off before you use the white block.

Q *220. How do I get a really high shine on my nails?*

A After you use the white block, buff with a three-way. Use the black side first, then the white side, and finally the gray side. Be sure to use enough pressure to be effective and use the entire file in long strokes for maximum coverage. The best buffing always comes from spending ample time perfecting each step.

Q *221. Can I use oil with a three-way high shiner?*

A Yes, but only on the coarse side. Otherwise you can ruin the file.

Q 222. *Is there a way to get a super high shine?*

A Yes, after you have gone through the steps of buffing you can use a chamois buffer with buffing creams. Or drop a small drop of acetone on the finest side of a three-way block buffer for a super shine.

Q 223. *How long does the shine last?*

A As long as the nails are not scratched with abrasives like Comet, it will last until the next fill.

Nail Notes

Nail Notes

Tip Application

Nail Tip Technology

Q *224. What are tips made of?*

A Most tips are made of ABS plastic that is durable and strong. Some are made of tenite acetate that are more flexible than the ABS plastic tips, but they don't stay on the nails as well as the ABS plastic ones do. Ninety-nine percent of the tips are made of ABS plastic.

One way to tell an ABS plastic tip from an tenite acetate tip is to bend the tip in half horizontally from side to side instead of down the middle of the tip from the cuticle to tip. The one that shows a white crease is the more flexible and is the tenite plastic.

Q *225. How are tips made?*

A Tips are made by injection molding with hot ABS or tenite acetate plastic material. Tips are molded on a tree-like form, and each tip is broken off the tree when cooled. That is why you may sometimes find a little glitch on the very tip if the tip is uneven. That is where it was attached to the tree.

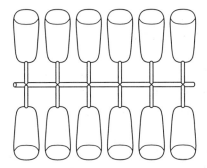

A tip tree.

Q *226. Where are tips made?*

A Years ago they were made overseas. But with the modern age of nail technology, we are finding more affordable equipment, and many American manufacturers are now making their own tips right in their warehouses.

Tip Fit & Design

Q *227. Who designs the tips?*

A Mostly the manufacturers and their technical advisors who are usually nail techs like you and me. Their designs are based on their experiences and needs at the salon.

Q *228. Why do tips fit differently?*

A Each tip manufacturer has its own unique design and can vary in shapes and sizes. Because not all nails are created equal, a variety of shapes are necessary to fit the variety of nails we see at the manicuring table.

Q 229. What is a tip well?

A The tip well is the contact area of the tip that actually fits on the nail plate. It is usually thinner than the rest of the tip for blending and flexibility purposes.

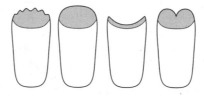

The shaded areas represent the tip wells.

Q 230. Why do some tips have bigger wells than others?

A Depending on the design, the shape can vary from tip to tip. Wells that are larger are for more coverage of the nail plate, and require more glue contact. A shorter well requires less glue contact. Some wells have v shapes, jagged edges, or very thin contact areas for blending purposes.

Q 231. What is the stop gap?

A Often called the contact point, it is the edge under the tip that the natural nail butts up against when the tip is applied. Before you apply the tip, file the natural nail to fit the

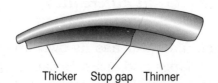

Thicker   Stop gap   Thinner

The stop gap is where the natural nail butts up against the division.

shape of the stop gap. Try the tip on before applying glue. When you turn the nail over, the natural nail should fit perfectly into the stop gap.

Q 232. *Why are most numbers located underneath?*

A So they can be blended with a little acetone or a polish corrector pen after you apply them. Some newer, more progressive tips have been manufactured with the numbers on the top side at the tip of the tips. This means you have to file and remove the numbers before you apply a product over them.

Tip Preparation

Q 233. *Should I pre-shape the tip before I apply it?*

A Yes, if you feel the fit would be better. However, it is not always necessary.

Q 234. *Where should I pre-shape?*

A You can pre-shape the sides if you feel the tip is a bit wide, or reshape the side walls for an arch as it extends from the nail groove. You can file the well area for a more blended look, or reshape it to fit the nail better.

Q 235. *What kind of files should I use to pre-shape the tips?*

A You can use any number of files to achieve this. A round disk file, a cushioned board or any medium grit file with flexibility can be used. You can also use an electric file or drill.

Q 236. *Do I need to blend the tip?*

A Not unless you plan to wear the tips without polish, and you cannot apply them invisibly. Some tips colors blend better than others, and you may consider that when choosing a tip. If you are going to polish the tips and it is not important what the nail looks like underneath, you can place the tip on the nail, cut and shape it, then apply product and finish the nail, all without ever filing or blending the tip.

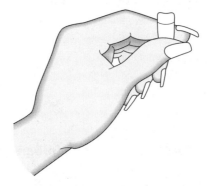

Hold the tip at an angle while filing.

Q 237. *What do I blend the tip with?*

A You can pre-file the tip well area before you apply the tip. This will prevent filing too much on the natural nail plate after you apply the tip.

You also can use a tip-blending product that is applied after the tip is glued on, and is left to soak into the tip. Let the blender sit on the well area for a minute or two; then take a coarse to medium file, and gently file off the melted product.

Another effective but more traditional way of blending the tip is to dip the tip well area into acetone just before applying the tip. This will soften and melt it a bit before application.

Q *238. When do I cut the tip?*

A You should cut the tip after it has been applied and is secure, and the glue has dried completely.

Q *239. What do I cut the tip with?*

A You may use a flat-sided large nail clipper or a tip clipper. The tip clipper will give you the most precise cut in one step while the nail clipper requires two cuts, one on each side of the tip. Then the cut is not smooth and must be filed.

Tip Application

Q *240. At what stage do I apply the tip?*

A Only after the natural nail has been prepared properly and dusted. Do not touch the nail plate at this point. You will only add natural oils from your fingers, which may promote lifting.

Q *241. What do I apply the tip with?*

A With a glue of your choice or in a ball of acrylic which is a glueless tip application.

Q *242. How do I apply the glue?*

A If you use a wet glue, place three small drops on the tip, one in the center and the other two on each side of the natural nail. Then turn the tip over and place three small drops of glue on the inside of the well as you did the natural nail.

If you use a thicker glue, draw a very thin line of glue along the tip of the natural nail and the under the edge of the tip well.

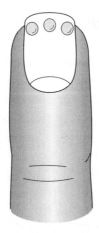

Glue application: Apply three dots of glue on nail at tip as shown.

Q **243. What if the glue dries before I can get the tip on?**

A If a glue dries before you can apply the tip, the glue is either setting too fast, or you are not applying the tip quick enough.

Q **244. How do I apply the tip?**

A After applying the glue, take the tip and fit the stop gap up against the natural free edge at a 90 degree angle. Gently press the tip so it meets the nail bed horizontally, evenly distributing the glue. Remove the tip in a wiping motion. Immediately repeat this procedure but do not remove the tip. Keep a little pressure on the tip until you feel the glue has dried enough to let go.

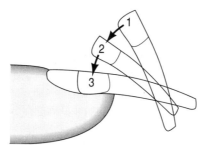

Tip application: Apply the tip at an angle and gently press the tip so that it meets the nail bed horizontally.

Q 245. What if I want to reposition the tip after I applied it?

A If you can manage to remove it before the glue sets, do so. But if the glue has dried too much, then soak the entire tip off in acetone and reapply a new tip.

Q 246. What if I used too much glue and it is under the tip of the nail?

A The client will feel a tightness if glue dries under the tip. When the glue is dry, have the client gently pull the skin away from the tip under the nail and break the seal. This may not be comfortable for the client until after her nail service. If you can, clean up the glue with an orangewood stick wrapped with some cotton and dipped in acetone, or use a polish corrector pen.

Q 247. Do I need to remove the glue that squeezed onto the nail plate when I pressed the tip on?

A If you plan on a natural look with little or no polish, I would remove it. The best time to do this is immediately after the tip application. With your finger, just wipe the wet glue off. If you choose to wait until the glue is dry, you can then file it off or use tip blender.

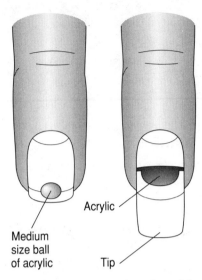

Medium
size ball
of acrylic

Acrylic

Tip

Apply a medium-sized ball of acrylic on the edge of the nail. Then, press the tip into the acrylic and hold it in position until dry.

Q *248. What if there are air bubbles in the glue?*

A There is no doubt about it, air bubbles in the glue weaken the tip application, so if you feel the need to re-apply, soak the nail off and do so. Proper wiping of the tip and distributing the glue evenly will prevent air bubbles in the glue.

Q *249. How do I apply a tip without glue?*

A Once the nail is prepared, you then prime the nail twice. Drop a small to medium ball of acrylic on the center of the tip of the natural nail and let it level off on its own. Once the acrylic starts to set up and the acrylic starts to look dull, press the tip into the acrylic and hold it in position until dry. This should take approximately 1 to 2 minutes.

Tip Adhesives

Q ***250. What are the different glues that can be used for tip application?***

A There are several types that are manufactured by several companies that range from very thin to thick or gellike. They are usually clear in color. Glues come in a variety of containers from brush-on applicators to large squeeze containers with tube necks for precise application, all usually with the same results.

Q ***251. What are the benefits of different glues?***

A Each can serve a different purpose, based on preference. A thin glue is good for a quick application or thin overlay for fiberglass mesh. A gel glue can serve as a filler for a tip application on a ridged nail. A very thin glue can be brushed onto the nail like polish giving extra support to a weak natural nail. A medium viscosity is your most common glue and used for most tip applications and breaks.

Q ***252. What is the average set-up time for glue?***

A Approximately a minute, depending on the viscosity. A thinner glue is going to set up quicker than a thicker glue.

Q ***253. Should I use a glue applicator?***

A Because they have long tubes, they can be helpful for a direct application and are easily replaceable when clogged up.

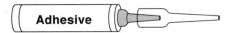

The tip applicator fits over the traditional glue container.

Q 254. How do I keep my glue from drying up?

A Always keep a lid on glue when it's not being used. Another trick is to replace the cap and tap the bottom of the bottle on the table, forcing the glue from the neck of the bottle back down.

Q 255. What can I do to speed up the glue process?

A You can always spray it with resin activator before or after application. Follow manufacturer's instructions and use a minimal amount of glue.

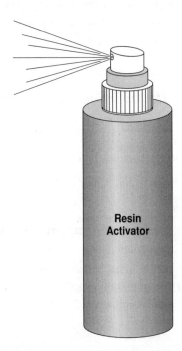

To speed up the glue process, spray the nail with resin activator.

Tip Removal

Q 256. When should I remove a tip?

A Usually when the tip has separated underneath, causing lifting between the tip of the natural nail and the end of the tip. Another reason would be for cosmetic purposes. A service that is growing in popularity is overlaying real white tips with a clear acrylic. Instead of backfilling the tips when the white grows out, you would remove them and replace the entire full set.

Q 257. How can I safely remove a tip?

A Soaking in non-acetone or straight acetone will melt the tips off. This process takes approximately 20 minutes for regular tips and 45 minutes for tips with an acrylic overlay. Be sure to wash the nails thoroughly and rehydrate them with a manicure or cuticle oil after the service. Be sure to pour the acetone into an acetone–proof bowl and dispose of the dirty acetone properly when done.

Q 258. Can I use tip blender to remove the tips?

A Yes, you can by filing the tip thin and applying tip blender. But you can do this only if there is a bare tip without an overlay.

Q 259. Should I cut the tip down first?

A This can help the removal process and make it neater in the long run.

Q 260. How do I apply a tip on a nail biter?

A It depends on the severity of the nail biting. You might want to build out the natural nail with a form, and then

apply an acrylic to the tip of the finger, shaping it into a natural looking nail. When the acrylic dries, shape the acrylic's
free edge to fit the tip well and smooth the top of it. Glue the
tip onto the acrylic's free edge, and cut and shape the tip.
Apply an acrylic overlay as usual.

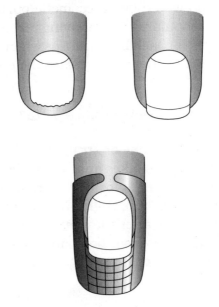

1: A bitten nail; 2: Using form and acrylic, extend the free edge over the finger; 3: Place the form over acrylic free edge and build a sculpted nail.

Q 261. How do I apply a tip on a ski jump nail?

A Shorten the free edge as much as you can during nail
preparation. Using a thick gel glue, apply a generous
amount to the tip of the free edge, and place the tip on the
nail. Do not press the tip to touch the entire nail plate. Instead, press the top edge of the well area touching the nail
and the rest into the glue until it gives you the profile you
would like. In other words, use the glue to fill in the gaps.
Wipe off any excess glue and let dry. Cut and shape the tip

and then overlay it with acrylic. Watch the profile as you apply so that you put on ample acrylic to fill in the dips where the contact area of the tip touches the natural nail.

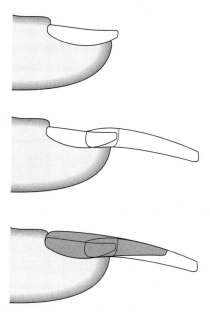

1: A ski jump nail; 2: Place the tip on the edge of the nail and use a glue gun or acrylic fill-in product to adhere the tip; 3: Fill in dips with acrylic and cut the tip. (The shaded area represents the final nail.)

Nail Notes

Nail Notes

Nail Wraps

Silk, Fiberglass & Linen

Q *262. What is the difference between silk, fiberglass and linen?*

A Each one of the different materials is slightly different from the other, all acting as reinforcements for the resin applied over them. Each one has its benefits, and it is a preference as to which one you choose.

Silk is the smoothest and thinnest. Because of the thinness, it practically disappears in the resin when applied properly. While it is just as strong as fiberglass, silk was the original material designed for use with resin. It usually comes without a self adhesive, and it is slightly more difficult to apply because of its silky texture.

Linen is more coarse and is not as popular because it is more difficult to blend into the resin. Fibers are bigger, although it too, provides good strength with the resin.

Fiberglass comes in various shades of pink and white. It usually comes with a sticky adhesive backing and is much more efficient. Strong and easy to use, it is almost invisible when applied properly and is very capable of making a beautiful, clear, natural-looking nail.

Q *263. What is the most common material used for wrapping nails?*

A Fiberglass, no doubt, is the most popular, then silk, followed by linen. Most resins are marketed with fiberglass or silk, but you can purchase materials elsewhere if you choose to.

Q *264. Do all materials come with self-adhesive?*

A No, they don't. However the more popular brands do come with self-adhesive on the back, with slick paper you peel off when applying. Some master technicians who have been performing this service for many years use a silk purchased at a material store and apply it without adhesive and get beautiful results. This is an art learned from many years of practice.

Q *265. What is the difference between the adhesives found on the back of the materials?*

A Thickness and quality. If you hold a piece of fiberglass up to the light, you can see the adhesive on the back. If it is bulky and very visible, it is an inexpensive piece of fiberglass and when applied, will not disappear into the resin very well. It will stay visible because of the adhesive, not the material.

Q *265. Do you need to use an overlay of resin with these wraps?*

A No, you don't, but the better you cover the material, the better the long term retention and wearability.

Q *266. Do I need to cut the wraps out?*

A Some wraps come pre-cut, but most of them come in a roll that you must cut yourself. Size and cut each piece to fit each nail plate. Keep a pair of sharp scissors just for cutting wrap material, and cut only what you need. Try not to touch the material with your fingers. Pick it up with tweezers or your nippers. The oils from your fingers can make the products lift.

Q 267. How do I apply the wraps?

A Step 1 Once the wrap is cut to fit, place over the nail and see if it overlaps any edges. If it does, trim the piece of material to fit without touching any edges of the nail. Leave approximately 1/16" of an inch around the cuticle and sidewalls exposed. Always hold the material with tweezers or your nippers when doing this. You should do two pieces of wrap material, one that covers most of the nail and the second to cover just enough over the stress area for reinforcement. You may also vary the angle of the mesh material for that added strength. Both pieces of wrap material can be applied one after the other or in between resin applications.

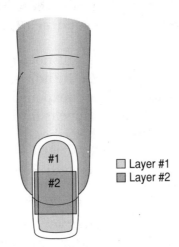

□ Layer #1
■ Layer #2

A fiberglass wrap.

Step 2 Before placing the material on the nail, lightly coat the nail with a thin layer of glue. The easiest way is to use a thin brush-on glue or a fast-setting thin glue in a tube. Put one coat on all ten nails. By the time you go back to the first nail to apply the mesh, it will be dry enough. This is a good way of getting silk without a self-adhesive back to stay on the nail.

Step 3 Once the wrap material has been applied, take an orangewood stick and pat out any ripples or spots that are not touching the nail itself.

Q 269. How do I apply the resin?

A The first coat on top of the wrap material should be a very thin and runny resin so it will quickly fill in all the nooks and crannies within the mesh. This is the secret to getting a clear looking wrap nail, no matter what materials and products you choose to use.

Step 1 Hold the nails at a downward angle. Starting in the center of the nail just below the cuticle, place a small drop of glue and let it run down the nail. With the tube on the glue, wipe from side to side for an even distribution. Or if you use a brush-on glue, brush over the entire nail with a thin resin until it has completely penetrated the material.

Step 2 Repeat this step two to three times, doing all ten nails with a thin resin or a thicker resin of your choice. Let the resin dry between coats if possible.

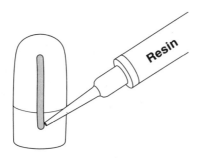

Resin application: Place a small drop of glue in the center of the nail and let it run down the nail.

Q 270. How do I cure the resin or does it dry on its own?

A When you have applied two to three coats of resin, with the activator, spray or apply all ten nails. Follow manufacturer's instructions on distance when spraying.

Q 271. Does the activator need to be wiped off the nails between applications?

A Yes, otherwise it will clog your resin applicator or dry the product on your brush. If that happens, replace the applicator and use a tip blender or soak the brush in eliminator.

Q 272. When do I file the nails?

A You can file the nails between each application if you choose to. If you have a smooth application, it will not be necessary until you have cured all the nails. However, for a finer finish, file and shape all the nails and apply one final coat of resin after you applied the activator. This will give you a finish that dries from the bottom up without the usual pitting. Be careful not to clog the applicator nozzle by using it at an angle when applying.

Q 273. Can the client wear the nails natural without polish?

A Yes, if you take extra care in application and blending the tips if you need extensions. Refer to sections on "Tip Application" (pages 99–102) and "Fill-Ins" (pages 161–175) for a more details on these steps.

Q 274. How do I get a shine on the nails?

A You actually have three options. You can perfect your skills so your final coat of resin is perfectly smooth and covered completely, so there are no flat spots, or you can buff to a high shine with a three-way buffer. (See the section on Buffing under "Filing and Shaping.") Or you can finish the nails with a super-shiny top coat.

Q *275. How does one remove overlays?*

A Fiberglass, silk, or linen wraps with resin overlays can be safely soaked off in acetone or non-acetone polish remover. Be sure to use a non-plastic dish, and plan on 20 to 30 minutes for the wraps to melt off.

Natural Nail Wrapping & Repairing

Q *276. What is the preferred wrap material for natural nails?*

A A fiberglass, silk, or linen wrap can easily be used in addition to a more traditional paper wrap. All are good options.

Q *277. Can you wrap natural nails and not damage them?*

A Yes you can. The product does not do the damage in this case; the technician does. The damage is in the work done during the application or fills. Clipping loose product, pulling an overlay off and overfilling or filing into the natural nail plate can all cause damage. This is not permanent damage, but is unnecessary. One must be extra cautious when working on the natural nails and take good care of them, because the purpose of the wrap is to enhance the natural nail, not replace or damage it.

Q *278. How do I apply wraps?*

A As you would any wrap. Refer to the previous section on "Silk, Fiberglass & Linen." Follow the same instructions for a tip and overlay wrap for natural nails.

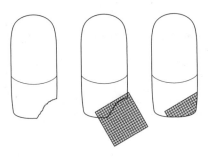

Fiberglass wrap repair

Q 279. Can you use any wrap material for repairing a natural nail?

A Yes, it is common to use a variety of products to repair a natural nail. It is gentler and kinder than an acrylic, and applied properly, can be strong and durable.

Q 280. Should you use glue with paper wraps?

A It is not necessary but can be done. Some techs mix a very thin glue with a clear polish and cover the paper wraps.

Q 281. What is a Juliette?

A It is a paper wrap, a thin paper material such as perm paper that can be wrapped on the nail and over the free edge of natural nails and covered with clear polish for added strength. Juliette is the name of the woman who invented the paper wrap.

Q 282. What other materials can you use for repairing natural nails?

A Cotton twisted and set in the crack itself with a touch of glue is an old standby. There are many new products that have come to market such as the vinyl adhesive that can be placed right over the polish and will hold the crack in a natural nail for weeks without damaging the nail.

Q 283. How do you remove the wraps?

A Paper wraps can be safely soaked off in acetone or non-acetone polish remover. Be sure to use a non-plastic dish, and plan on 10 to 15 minutes for paper wraps to dissolve. If there is a resin overlay they may take a few more minutes.

Q 284. What is the maintenance on wrapping natural nails?

A Every two to three weeks with a maintenance manicure between visits is suggested.

Tip Overlay Wrapping

Q 285. What is the procedure for wrapping a tip and overlay?

A It is the same as a regular wrap as we have addressed in the previous chapters with the extension applied before the wrap. If the client needs a more natural look, the tip should be blended before the mesh is applied. It is not necessary to wrap the mesh under the tips.

Q 286. Can silk, fiberglass, or linen be used?

A Yes, your preference on what you choose to work withdepends on the needed strength, the finished look you want to achieve, and the performance of the wrap material itself.

Q *287. What should be used to overlay the wrap?*

A Resin, as we addressed earlier. However the longer the extension, the more wrap product and extra layers of resin you may want to apply for a stronger seal on the nail.

Q *288. How many layers of glue and material is suggested?*

A For a medium-length extension, it is suggested that two pieces of mesh material be used: one covering 85 percent of the nail and the other 50 percent, and centered in the middle. If you feel it is necessary for a third, place it across the stress area. Several layers of resin are also suggested: one or two thin layers and two to three thicker layers over the top.

Q *289. With the extra layers of resin will the nails get hot when I use the activator? What do I do if it does?*

A If the nails get hot, the problem is too much resin, not enough or too much activator. You might want to split the activating up into two or three applications, activating as you go. If the nails get hot, immediately spray them again or immerse them in cool water. Then re-evaluate your application and reread your manufacturer's instructions. You may be spraying too close or too far away.

Q *290. What causes the resin to get hot?*

A The product scrambling to dry because the resin to activator ratio was not equal. As soon as you spray the hot nails again, the product is dry and cools right off.

Liquid Nail Wrapping

Q *291. What is a liquid wrap?*

A It is a denser polish product similar to ridge filler with actual synthetic fibers in it to strengthen the natural nails when dry. It is usually a gray or white color, dries more slowly than the average polish, and can look a bit rough on the surface when the fibers show through. This is sometimes referred to as a "liquid Juliette."

Q *292. Who makes this product?*

A Several companies make their own version of liquid wraps, mainly the natural nail care companies.

Q *293. Should you apply more than one layer of liquid wrap?*

A Two layers is suggested for maximum strength.

Q *294. Should you let each layer dry between coats?*

A Absolutely. One of the frustrations of using this product is the need for ample drying time between coats of polish, especially liquid wrap products.

Q *295. When done polishing, how many coats of polish will the client actually have applied?*

A If the client wants to wear a color, the total will be 5 or 6 depending on whether you need to use a base coat over the liquid wrap. There are two coats of liquid wraps, two coats of color, and one top coat. Ultraviolet lights can assist in the drying process and should be used after each coat of polish.

Ridge filler can be used in place of the base coat and over the liquid wrap products, or in addition to the base coat. I would recommend using only one coat because the liquid wrap can be as thick as the ridge filler.

Nail Preparation

Q *296. Is it necessary to take any extra steps in preparing the natural nails before any silk, fiberglass, linen, or liquid wrap services?*

A Yes, a basic manicure. Or you should clean the natural nail plate, pushing the cuticles back, and reshape the natural free edges before application.

Q *297. Do I need to put any dehydrators or chemicals on the natural nails to change or balance the condition of the nails?*

A No. Primers should never be used. However nail preparation products that are part of the systems you are using can be used.

Maintenance

Q *298. How often is it necessary to reapply or maintain nails wearing liquid wraps?*

A For a natural nail liquid wrap, a weekly manicure is suggested for maximum results. Start by removing the polish and liquid wrap products with non-acetone or acetone polish removers. Perform a complete natural nail care manicure and reapply the liquid wrap material before applying colors.

Q *299. How often is it necessary to maintain fill-ins with fiberglass, silk, or linen?*

A For a fiberglass, silk, or linen wrap, maintenance should be approximately two to three weeks depending on the client's care and how she wears them. Use your judgment and professional knowledge and advise your client when she should see you, depending on how her nails hold up.

Q *300. What is the application time for fiberglass, silk, or linen wrap fill-ins?*

A The application time for a fiberglass, silk, or linen wrap fill-in should be approximately 45 minutes to 1 hour.

Step 1 Start by removing the polish and pushing the cuticles back.

Step 2 File any lifting around the cuticle area flush with the natural nail with a medium or coarse file. File the sides and the tips of the nails where the seal of resin has been broken. File a ridge into any cracks that may need fixing.

Step 3 File the top layer of the entire nail and reshape all 10 nails. Shorten if necessary.

Step 4 Brush the dust off the nails with a nylon brush.

Step 5 Reapply the resin as directed in the previous section on fiberglass application.

Nail Notes

Acrylic Extensions

Nail Preparation

Q *301. What do I need to do to the natural nails in preparation for an acrylic overlay or sculptured nail?*

A A series of steps to properly prepare the natural nails are important.

Step 1 Push the cuticles back and remove all ptergyium.

Step 2 Shape natural nails.

Step 3 Gently buff the top of the nail plate with a soft file to remove the shiny surface.

Step 4 Dust nail plate with nylon brush.

Step 5 Dehydrate the nail plate.

Step 6 Prime the nails.

Q *302. Should I use a sanitation spray on the nails?*

A No! Sanitation sprays are for the hands before you start your services, not on the nail plate after you have prepared the nails.

Q 303. Should I use a dehydrator?

A Yes, after the nail is prepared and dusted, and before the primer is the correct time to use a dehydrator.

Q 304. What is the purpose of using a dehydrator?

A A dehydrator is used to dehydrate the nail plate, removing all the moisture for better retention. There are dehydrators that are stronger than others, so use your common sense when using a dehydrator.

Q 305. Do I have to use a dehydrator?

A No, this is an option and should not be used if the nails are already very dry.

Q 306. When do I prime the nails?

A After the dusting of the nail plate and use of the dehydrator.

Tip & Overlay

Q 307. What is an acrylic tip and overlay?

A An acrylic tip and overlay is a plastic tip applied to the natural nail. An acrylic overlay that is applied over the entire natural nail and extension provides strength and durability to the tip.

Q *308. What determines the use of a tip and overlay versus a sculptured nail?*

A Base the use of the tip and overlay on two things. Preference is one reason. Some techs prefer to do a tip and overlay rather that a sculptured nail for personal reasons. The other reason is cosmetic. The shape of the nail, the length of free edges, and ease of use of the tip should determine whether you use a tip and overlay.

Q *309. Can I make the tip and overlay look like a sculptured nail?*

A Absolutely. Today's tip manufacturers have created enough different types, colors, and styles to choose from that will give you enough diversity to match any sculptured nail.

Q *310. Are tips and acrylic overlays stronger?*

A Yes and no. Technically, if a tip and overlay are correctly applied and a sculptured nail is correctly sculpted on a nail with enough free edge for support, both can be equally strong. Unfortunately, the conditions on every nail, tip and overlay, or sculptured nail are not always perfect, and you must call on your professional experience to determine what you will use.

Sculptured Nail

Q *311. What is a sculptured nail?*

A A sculptured nail is the application of acrylic over the natural nail that is extended with the support of a form under the free edge of the natural nail.

Q *312. What kind of forms are needed to sculpt nails?*

A Forms come in several shapes and sizes in paper, plastic, and metal materials. Some have different thickness for durability. They can be dual sided and designed for specific fingers, or one size fits all. Some are reusable and some are throw aways. The choice is up to the technician.

Q *313. Is a sculptured nail the right service for every client?*

A No, not always. Assessing the right service for the client is part of our professional responsibility and knowing when to sculpt and not to sculpt is important. Nail biters, nails without ample free edge, wide or ski jump nails where the forms do not fit well under the free edge are all candidates for other services. There should be some free edge and a nail bed in good shape to consider sculpting. There should be corners on the free edge to catch the form underneath. The free edge can assist in supporting the sculpted extension.

Q *314. Can a sculptured nail offer the same strength as a tip and overlay?*

A When properly applied under the correct conditions, yes it can.

Q *315. At what length can you comfortably sculpt a set of long nails without any breakage?*

A The key here is balance. You don't want the tip of the extension to be top heavy and longer than the nail bed itself. A safe and suggested length that can easily be supported is one-half the length of the natural nail or shorter.

Q *316. How long does it take to sculpt a full set of nails?*

A The average time for a new set of sculptured nails is 60 to 90 minutes, depending on how experienced you are.

Q *317. What is the recommended maintenance?*

A Every two to three weeks, depending on the client's wear ability.

Traditional Acrylic Products

Q *318. What is a traditional acrylic?*

A A traditional acrylic is a mix of liquid monomer and acrylic powder, which when mixed is applied with a brush over the nails and that hardens to a surface that can be filed and shaped.

Q *319. How long have acrylics actually been a nail service?*

A For more than 30 years. Developed from dental products and manufactured mostly in the Los Angeles area, acrylics still remain the leading artificial nail service nationwide.

Q *320. What is a slow- or medium-set acrylic?*

A Most of the original acrylics that have been around a long time were developed with a slow or medium set-up time of 2–3 minutes. This product is easier to use for the novice technician.

Q *321. What is a fast-set acrylic?*

A A fast set is an acrylic formulation that sets up quicker than the traditional acrylic products first introduced to the nail market. The faster set products are for the more seasoned technicians.

Q *322. What colors do acrylics come in?*

A Colors vary from company to company but the general versions are white for tips, clear, pink or peach for the base of the nails, and natural for one-color nails.

Q *323. Do the colors change the chemical makeup of the product?*

A No. Although the density may appear to be different, the workability remains the same.

Q *324. What is the recommended maintenance?*

A Every two to three weeks, depending on the client's wear ability.

Light-Activated Acrylic Nails

Q *325. What exactly is a light-activated acrylic?*

A The ingredients are generally the same, however the catalyst is a light-activated chemical that reacts to ultraviolet light.

Q *326. What kind of light is needed?*

A A compatible ultraviolet lamp designed by the acrylic manufacturer to work with the acrylic. Wattage is approximately 4 watts per bulb.

Q *327. How long does it take for the nails to set up?*

A Approximately the same time as a traditional acrylic, 2 minutes if used with a dryer consistency, more if a wetter consistency is used.

Q *328. Can I sculpt with forms or do I need to overlay tips?*

A It is very difficult to sculpt with a light-activated acrylic, and using a tip and overlay technique will probably give you much better results.

Q *329. What are the benefits of using a light-activated acrylic?*

A This is an odorless product and allows the technician to work in a fresher environment while providing the clients the same benefit.

Q *330. How are they different from traditional acrylics?*

A Workability is different and you must work with a drier consistency than with a traditional acrylic. The liquid to powder ratio requires less liquid and needs some practice to achieve the right consistency.

Q *331. What are the drawbacks?*

A A sticky residue is left on top of the nail after it cures and must be removed by filing before you can file and shape the entire nail.

Q *332. What is the recommended maintenance?*

A Every two to three weeks, depending on the client's wear ability.

Odorless Acrylic

Q *333. What is odorless acrylic?*

A It is an acrylic product with odorless ingredients that has a slower evaporation and makes the smell less noticeable than traditional acrylics.

Q *334. How is it different from traditional acrylic and light-activated acrylic?*

A The chemistry and application is similar to the traditional acrylics. However, the technical set-up is different and more similar to the gels. The thicker the product, the slower the set up.

Q *335. Are the odorless acrylics really safer to use?*

A I am not sure that any one product is safer to use than any other. However, the odorless products have definite benefits to the salon and technician by providing an environment that does not smell like acrylics.

Q *336. Are odorless acrylics as good as traditional acrylics?*

A This depends on the usage and the technician's ability to apply them. A good tech can apply any product well for good results.

Problem Nails

Q *337. How do I apply acrylic nails to wide nails?*

A The best answer to this is to use a wide tip and overlay. However, we sometimes run into a nail that is wider than the tips that are available. In that case, what you want to do, is sculpt a nail with a modified form.

Take two forms and cut off the opposite sides of each form and stick them together. Cut the inside of the form smooth and to the desired shape, and you have created a custom form for that wide nail.

Q *338. How do I apply nails to a nail biter who has skin on the tips of her fingers that is higher than the nail beds?*

A The best bet is to ask the client to be patient and do the extensions in two parts. First overlay her natural nails with clear acrylic and let them grow for approximately one month, so the natural nails extend over the skin. This allows the skin to recede naturally, and gets the nails to grow and the client accustomed to not biting her nails. Once the acrylic overlay resembles a natural nail that is not bitten and has grown a small free edge, fill the acrylic in as usual. To extend the nails, place a form under the free edge and sculpt the nail as usual. If you prefer a tip and overlay, apply the tip with wet acrylic instead of glue, and proceed with the process of a tip and overlay as usual.

Q *339. How do I repair an acrylic nail that is cracked across the nail bed?*

A First, with a drill of an electric file, bevel both sides of the crack almost flush with the natural nail. Glue the crack and wipe off the excess glue. Apply acrylic into the beveled area and file flush with the remainder of the nail. It is not necessary to prime the cracked area.

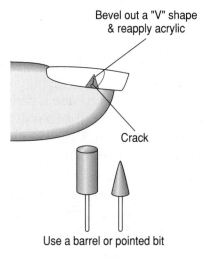

Repairing an acrylic nail that is cracked across the nail bed

Q *340. Should I recommend that a client glue a nail that has lifted?*

A Yes, if you feel the client can apply the glue properly. Sparingly, is the best way to apply glue just around the cuticle area while holding the nail at an angle so the glue flows right into the lifting area. If a client has consistent lifting, you need to reconsider her service or identify why she is lifting.

Educating the client on how to use the glue properly can help the glue application's longevity. Don't just sell her the glue; explain how to keep the neck of the glue container clean by wiping it after each use, by using only a drop at a time, and holding the container at an angle to properly receive the glue. Explain to her that she should make sure the nail is dry before gluing it.

Q *341. How do I correct a crooked natural nail?*

A First, remove all acrylic from the nail and shorten the natural nail as much as possible, leaving a small free edge. Whether you choose to do an acrylic tip and overlay or a sculptured nail, the trick to applying it straight is to look at the overall nail and finger when applying it. If you extend the nail and only look at the nail bed when applying, you are only extending the crooked nail so it starts at the cuticle, not fixing the direction of the entire nail. You must look at the whole finger when applying the nail.

Be sure to look down the barrel of the nail as you apply. Sometimes you may need to adjust the application to the top of the nail to compensate for its crooked placement on the natural nail.

You may get the nail to look straight but within fills, the nails can reassume their crooked growth pattern. You may need to be replace it each time you fill the client to keep it straight.

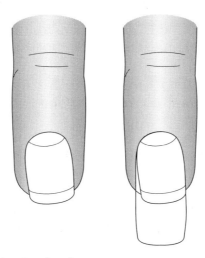

Correcting a crooked natural nail.

Chemical Reactions to Liquid & Powder Nails

Q 342. What exactly causes a chemical reaction?

A Usually overexposure or sensitivity. Redheads or extremely fair clients with thin skin may have a reaction sooner than the average client. A client who works in a dental office and is exposed to dental-making products may be overexposed.

Another way of over exposing the client is to touch the surrounding skin with the products you are using, such as primer and liquid monomer. It is very important that you do not touch the skin with these chemicals.

Q 343. What does a technician look for in a reaction?

A Red, swollen, itchy cuticles.

Q 344. What exactly is causing the reaction?

A Allergic reactions are most likely due to the liquid component of the product, which is why you should be extremely careful not to get primers and liquids on the skin surrounding the nails.

Q 345. How long after the client has her nails done should she see a reaction if she is allergic?

A Two or three days after the service is the average time for an allergic reaction to surface.

Q 346. What can be done to avoid reactions?

A Remove the nails and condition the cuticles with cuticle oils and conditioners.

Q *347. Once a client has a reaction can she ever wear the products again?*

A In time, she may be able to, but realistically you should try other products with different chemical compounds. It is not uncommon for a client to always react to the product no matter how long she waits.

Q *348. If the client can wear the products that gave her the reaction, how much time should she wait before reapplying the products?*

A I would wait several months. Try applying one nail and have the client check for any reaction before you attempt to reapply the product on all ten nails.

Q *349. If the nails need to be removed and the cuticles are red and swollen, how do you care for the nails without irritating the client's fingers more?*

A Apply a generous amount of petroleum jelly on her cuticles and soak the product off in acetone. Acetone is harsh but is the quickest. If the client is too sensitive, gently file the product off.

Q *350. Can I become allergic to any products?*

A Yes, and it is not uncommon. Barrier creams, gloves, and washing hands and arms thoroughly between clients can help alleviate the reactions.

Form Fitting

Q *351. What kind of form do you suggest the novice technician use for the best fit?*

A A traditional paper form shaped in a large "U." The key to a good form is the durability and thickness of the paper and the adhesive quality of the glue on the back that prevents it from moving once it has been applied. Most forms come with lines for building the nails straight and the same length. Some even have numbers on the lines.

Q 352. *Are there different kinds of forms for different nails?*

A Yes, many to choose from. All manufacturers that sell forms have designed their own version, each unique. The holes or the inside of the "U" can vary dramatically and should be the deciding factor on the proper fit. Be sure to note the shape upon purchase.

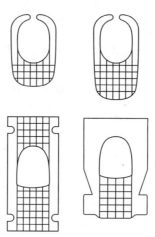

Paper forms.

Q 353. *How are metal forms different from paper forms?*

A Metal forms can vary like paper forms do. Thickness, plain or lined, different inside shapes, as well as parameter shapes are all variables.

Q 354. *Can all forms be reused?*

A Metal forms are reusable and paper forms are disposable.

Q **355. Do all forms come with lines on them?**

A Not all of them do. Both paper and metal forms are manufactured with and without lines. A little trick I have
learned is to apply a lined paper form over an unlined metal
form. This gives the technician the best of both worlds.

Q **356. How do you shape a metal form?**

A Wrap the metal form around a dowel to preshape it.
Dowels vary in size and are usually made of wood.

Q **357. How does one reuse a metal form and does it
need to be cleaned?**

A Once the metal form is removed, place it on your table.
Rub the flat end of the dowel over the form, removing
any acrylic residue while flattening it for the next use. If you
feel the need to clean the form better, soaking it in acetone
will remove any leftover acrylic. Metal forms can be sanitized,
too.

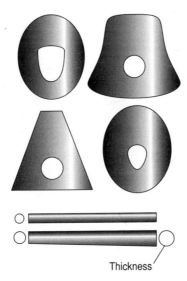

Metal forms and dowels.

Q **358. How do you know if the form is on correctly and won't slip?**

A When you start to apply acrylic, the form can shift, so you must be sure that it is on tightly. First, ask the client if it feels secure. Second, you can pinch the tip of a long form together for additional support at the sides of the nail at the stress area. With your thumbs, pinch in and make dents on the sides of the forms for better security.

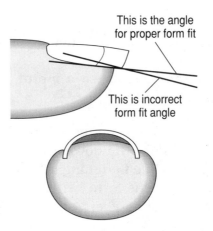

Fitting the form. 1: The correct angle for properly fitting a form. 2: The shaded area shows thick acrylic that will produce a big ridge when grown out. This happened because the form was improperly placed under the natural nail.

Q **359. What do you do if the form fits too snugly under the natural nail and pinches the client?**

A Replace the form. Do not attempt to pull it out. This only makes the client feel comfortable temporarily. Once you start applying the acrylic, the form will tighten and make the client even more uncomfortable.

Q **360. What is a c-curve?**

A It is the convex and concave c-shape of the nail extension that you see when looking down the barrel of the nail.

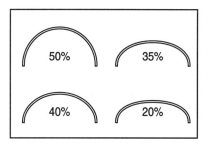

C-curves.

Q *361. How do you make a deep c-curve with a form?*

A If you use a metal form, you can preshape the c-curve with a small dowel before you apply the form. If you choose to use a paper form, wait until the acrylic is applied and it starts to dry. With the tops of your thumbnails pressed to the sides of the nail, press until you reach the desired c-shape and hold until the nail has dried permanently.

Application Structure

Q *362. What is the most important technique in applying liquid and powder acrylic?*

A Understanding the liquid to powder ratio with every stroke will give you the control you need for a precise application.

Q *363. Should I wet the natural nail plate with liquid monomer before I apply the acrylic?*

A You can, however this is not necessary. Some technicians have better retention when they wet the nail bed with liquid from their sculpting brush. If this works for you, then I recommend that you incorporate this procedure. However, if you do not see better results, then it is not necessary.

Q **364. How do I control the ratio of liquid to powder in my brush?**

A By controlling the amount of liquid you pick up in your brush even before you pick up acrylic. Here are some hints:

- Always use fresh, clean liquid for each client.
- Wipe your brush against the side of your dappan dish on its way out of the dish.
- Use a dappan dish that doesn't slide, so when you wipe your brush you have more control.
- Touch the tip of the brush on your table towel to remove the excess liquid.

Your liquid to powder ratio for an average ball of products should be 1 part liquid to two parts powder. Understanding this and adjusting the ratio for a wetter or dryer ball is the trick to controlling you application.

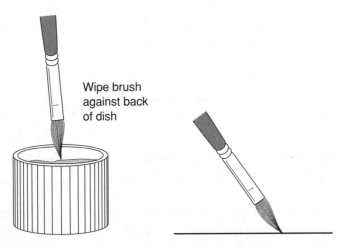

Wipe brush
against back
of dish

To control the ratio of liquid to powder acrylic on your brush, wipe the brush against the side of the dappan dish. Then, touch the tip on your table towel to remove excess liquid.

Q *365. Which is the best way to pick up the acrylic on my brush?*

A Do not submerge the tip of your brush into the powder. Gently, with the tip, press into the powder two or three times to get the ball you desire. Another way is to gently drag or wipe the brush, or make a small circle with the tip.

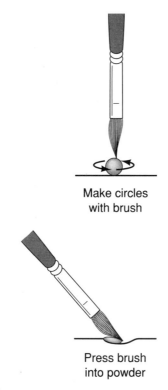

Make circles
with brush

Press brush
into powder

What is the best way to pick up acrylic with my brush?

Q *366. What happens if the product starts drying in my brush?*

A You must immediately wipe your brush and submerge it into the liquid until all the acrylic in the brush dissolves. There could be two problems here: 1. You are not getting the product off the brush fast enough when applying or 2. You are not wiping your brush immediately after dropping the product onto the nail before patting into place.

Q **367. Is there a pattern to applying acrylic?**

A Yes, there are a couple with different zones and specific applications for each zone.

Q **368. What is the most common way of applying?**

A Zone 1, Zone 2, and Zone 3.

Zone 1 is the tip of the nail. Usually a larger, drier ball of acrylic is applied. The drier the product, the tighter the cross linkage, the stronger the tip.

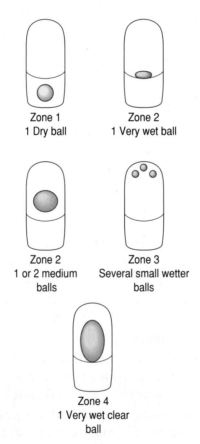

Zone 1
1 Dry ball

Zone 2
1 Very wet ball

Zone 2
1 or 2 medium
balls

Zone 3
Several small wetter
balls

Zone 4
1 Very wet clear
ball

The most common ways of applying acrylic.

Zone 2 is the center of the nail. It should be 1 or 2 medium-size balls of a wetter consistency, for more flexibility.

Zone 3, is the cuticle area. Several smaller balls of product, much wetter for good retention and smooth application that flows into the cuticle area with maximum flexibility .

Q *369. What is another way of application?*

A Following the specific directions for each zone as stated above, apply Zone 1 then apply Zone 3, and finally Zone 2.

Q *370. What is two-toning?*

A "Two-toning" or "pink and white" nails is the use of two separate acrylic colors to achieve a permanent French manicure look. Pink, peach, clear, and white tip powders can be used.

Q *371. How do you prevent dragging the pink acrylic through the white product?*

A Let the white tip powder dry until it looks dull before you apply Zone 2. This way you don't disturb the smile line or drag the pink through it. Another trick is to apply the white tip high enough, so you do not have to apply pink over it.

Q *372. What is a smile line?*

A A smile line is the natural distinction between the nail bed and the free edge of a natural nail. It is commonly referred to when sculpting pink and white acrylic nails. The white tip acrylic is applied and formed below and up to the natural smile line. The actual division is wiped in a perfect

"U" to resemble the natural smile line, before the rest of the clear or pink acrylic is applied.

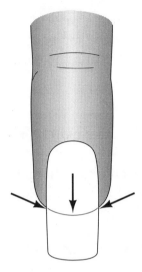

A smile line is the natural distinction between the nail bed and the free edge of the natural nail.

Troubleshooting

Q *373. What are air bubbles?*

A Air bubbles are caused by anything from excess air in your sculpting brush to a warm and humid environment. You will find that air bubbles happen mostly with faster setting liquid and powder systems, and in larger application balls of product. The air bubbles are more prominent in the Zone 2 area of the nails, over the stress areas.

Q *374. Can air bubbles affect the nails?*

A Yes they can. If a nail has a lot of air bubbles, which are air pockets, they will break when filed and look like tiny craters. These air pockets weaken the nail where it needs the most strength. The open air bubble when exposed can collect dirt and makeup, making the nails look like they have tiny black spots, a flaw when the client wears her nails buffed.

Q 375. *How can you get rid of air bubbles?*

A Proper liquid to powder ratios and application techniques can help you understand how to create nails free of air bubbles. A wetter, smaller, slower application in Zone 2 can help. Using a product that flows easily for you can also help.

Q 376. *What makes acrylic nail hot?*

A A quick application makes for a quick set up. A fast-set product is more likely to make a nail hot because it sets quickly. Pulling the form off immediately serves as an oven for the heat. Thumbs and middle nails are bigger so they are more susceptible to getting hot.

If you are having problems with heat but like the product, you can change your procedures by splitting the application into sections. Start by applying the tip on the pinky, then go to the ring finger. Go back to the pinky and apply Zone 2, then go to the middle nail and apply the tip. Go to the ring finger and apply Zone 2, then Zone 3 on the pinky. And so on. Splitting up the drying process can head off the heat.

Q 377. *What do I do when the nail is hot and the client complains?*

A Some techs pour alcohol over it or spray it with water. I take the heal of my hand and press it against the hot nail and draw the heat out. By the time the client mentions that the nail is hot, it is already starting to cool down. Sensitive and thin nails will feel the heat more.

Q 378. Why do acrylic nails turn yellow?

A Most of the time, if the acrylic turns yellow, it is because it is not a progressive product. Filling over top coat, sunscreens, and tanning products can also contribute.

Q 379. What do I do if there is a large pocket in the center of the nail that has lifted but the outside edges are still adhered?

A File the lifting area in the center of the nail down to the natural nail. Reprime and reapply the acrylic.

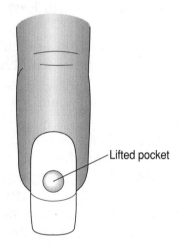

Lifted pocket

A large pocket in the center of the nail. File the area down to the natural nail, reprime, and reapply the acrylic.

Nail Notes

Gel Nails

Nail Preparation

Q **380. What do I need to do to the natural nails in preparation for a gel application?**

A A series of steps to properly prepare the natural nails are important.

Step 1 Push the cuticles back and remove all pterygium.

Step 2 Shape natural nails.

Step 3 Gently buff the top of the nail plate with a soft file to remove the shiny surface.

Step 4 Dust nail plate with nylon brush.

Step 5 Dehydrate the nail plate.

Q **381. Should I use a sanitation spray on the nails?**

A No! Sanitation sprays are for the hands before you start your services, not on the nail plate after you have prepared the nails.

Q 382. Should I use a dehydrator?

A Yes, you can. The proper time to use a dehydrator is after the nail is prepared and dusted, and before the primer.

Q 383. Do I have to use a dehydrator?

A No, this is an option and should not be used if the nails are already very dry.

Q 384. Do I need to use a primer?

A Most gel manufacturers claim that you do not need to use a primer when applying gel nails and you should first follow the manufacturer's instructions. Primers can be used if necessary.

Gel Applications

Q 385. What is a light cured gel?

A A gel is an acrylic product that has a honey-like sticky viscosity. Gels have a photo initiator chemical that sets or hardens the product when put under an ultraviolet lamp.

Q 386. What is a no-light gel?

A A no-light gel is a cyanoacrylate product, the same as that in your fiberglass resin products. Cyanoacrylate is an adhesive that is made thicker to gel-like consistency and marketed as a no-light gel.

Q 387. How are gels different from acrylics?

A In workability and wearability. However they are similar in chemical makeup. The major difference is in the catalysts. Acrylics have a catalyst in the liquid and powders that when mixed, start to set up. The gels have to be cured under a light and react to the photo initiator in the gel.

Q 388. What are the benefits of gels?

A They are definitely an alternative to liquid and powders, and fiberglass nails, providing 75 percent of the strength of an acrylic with the thinness of the fiberglass. They are less damaging than the acrylics, odorless, need almost no filing, and are easier to apply.

Q 389. What is the wattage of the lights used to cure gels?

A Usually the wattage varies from 4-watt bulbs to 8-watt bulbs, depending on the manufacturer of the light.

Q 390. Can you use a gel from one company and a light from another?

A Only if the wattage is identical. However the manufacturer will not guarantee its product if not used with the entire system. But the results can be the same if the wattage is the same. One way to tell if the light is wrong is when the gel will not set up correctly. It will remain sticky and dull.

Q 391. What kind of brush do I need to use?

A A synthetic square or slightly oval, but short brush is needed. A sable brush will only absorb the gel and make it difficult to apply.

Q 392. *How is the product applied?*

A There are several ways of applying, depending on the container and viscosity of the products. Some come in a squeeze bottle and some in a small container, from which you need to scoop the gel out with your brush. The choice is yours.

Some manufactures have a thin base gel, a thicker builder gel and a shiny sealer gel, all made of the same products, just a different viscosity. Some are made with one viscosity where you apply several coats. The choice is yours. Application is basically the same no matter what type of a gel you prefer.

Step 1 Prepare the nails by shaping and pushing the cuticles back.

Step 2 Buff the natural nail plate gently to remove the shine only.

Step 3 Dust the nail plate with a nylon brush.

Step 4 Apply nail dehydrator or nail preparation products.

Step 5 One hand at a time, apply 1 coat of gel, a thin base gel or the first coat of a one-gel system. Place the gel in the center of the nail plate just below the cuticle. With your brush, gently wipe the gel down the center of the nail plate. Then wipe on either side of the original gel application to each side of the nail, covering the entire nail. Wipe the little bit that is left on the brush against the three edges of the nail tip to seal the edges.

Step 6 Cure the nails for the manufacturer's suggested time. The curing time can vary from manufacturer to manufacturer.

Step 7 To keep the product from running to one side, you may want to apply the ring, middle and index fingers first, then the pinky and thumb. This will keep the product more centered on the nails before going under the light.

Another technique is to do the thumbs together, then cure them completely before applying the other 8 nails. Whatever system you decide on, stick to it. Jumping around will only waste time.

Step 8 Repeat step 5 with the second coat of gel or the builder gel and cure.

Step 9 Repeat step 8 with the final coat of gel and cure.

Q *393. Do I wipe the sticky layer off between coats of gel?*

A No, it is necessary to leave it on for better adhesion. However you must remove it from the top layer.

Q *394. What do I remove the sticky layer with?*

A Use a manufacturer gel wipe. If you use alcohol, it will leave the nails dull.

Q *395. How do I remove the gel I got on my client's cuticle?*

A Use the gel wipe and a polish corrector pen.

Q *396. My clients experience some stinging at first. What is this attributed to?*

A This is the gel drying process and usually happens on sensitive nails, virgin nails, or on a nail where the product has replaced the nail. This usually happens when they first place their nails in the light.

Q *397. What do I do for the stinging?*

A Have the client briefly remove her hand from the light and slowly put the nails back under the light. You slow down the drying process by removing the nails for approximately 10 seconds.

Q *398. Do I need to file the nails?*

A No, but this is optional. The simplicity of gel application is definitely a benefit, and if you can apply the gels smoothly enough without any lumps or bumps, it is not necessary to file. However if you feel the need, remove the sticky layer with gel wipe and gently file or buff the shape. Wipe the nail clean and reapply the gel.

Q *399. Can I polish the nails without ruining the shine?*

A Yes, you can. Polish does not hurt the shiny finish and if your client wishes to remove her polish between visits, the shine will still be there after she removes the polish.

Q *400. Can my clients wear the gels with out polish?*

A Yes, the shiny finish makes for a perfect finish. However some gels absorb discoloration when not protected with a top coat. The discoloration is just on the surface and can easily be removed by buffing.

Q *401. How do you remove gels?*

A You can safely and quickly remove gels by soaking them in acetone. This softens and separates the gel overlay so you can remove the overlay in one piece. It does not melt like acrylics. Older traditional gels need to be filed off.

Natural Nails

Q *402. Can I use gels over natural nails?*

A Yes, this is definitely a perfect way to enhance the natural nails without damage from other artificial products. The finished look of a gel can look as natural as a clear coat of polish on a natural nail.

Q *403. What is the benefit of gel as opposed to using a tip and overlay?*

A It depends on the length you desire. If your client wants help in growing her natural nails this is the perfect solution. With products on her natural nails, they will grow faster and protect her cuticles. Maintenance with fill-in will also stimulate their growth, and within a month or two she will have some length to her natural nails without the damage of tip overlays.

Q *404. Should I coat the underside of the natural nails with gel?*

A Yes you can. This not only seals the natural free edges of the nails, it provides additional strength to the nails.

Q *405. What is the recommended maintenance?*

A Every two to three weeks. See the section for "Fill-ins" on page 161.

Tip & Overlays

Q *406. What is a gel tip and overlay?*

A A gel tip and overlay is a plastic tip applied to the entire natural nail and extension, providing strength and durability to the tip.

Q *407. Can I make the gel tip and overlay look like a natural nail?*

A Absolutely. Today's tip manufacturers have created enough different types, colors and styles to give you enough diversity to match any natural nail.

Q *408. Are tips and gel overlays stronger than acrylic?*

A No, but technically, if a gel tip and overlay is correctly applied, it can be almost as strong.

Sculptured Gel Nails

Q *409. How are the gels sculptured?*

A Sculpting gels is tricky and you need a paper or metal form. See the section on "Form Fitting" on page 135. This is not a popular procedure.

Step 1 With a builder gel, apply the gel on the free edge over the form. Cure for approximately 1 minute, then remove.

Step 2 Reshape the parameter of the gel with your application brush. Reapply the gel, then cure for the full amount of time.

Step 3 Apply a base gel on the natural nail and cure.

Step 4 Apply two to three coats of builder gel over the entire nail and cure between each layer.

Refer to the "Gel Application" section on page 149.

Q 410. Do you need to file them?

A No it is not necessary but it is always an option if there is a need.

Q 411. How long can you sculpt the gel nails?

A The shorter the stronger. However the client's wearability and length of her free edge will determine a safe length.

Q 412. What is the maintenance on sculptured gels?

A Maintenance is just the same as with a traditional sculptured nail.

Repairs

Q 413. How do I repair a gel nail?

A If the nail is broken off and you need to replace the entire tip, you should remove all the gel by filing it flush with the natural nail. Replace it completely following the instructions in the "Gel Application" section on page 149.

Q 414. How do I repair a crack in the free edge of the natural nail?

A At an angle, bevel with a file into the crack until you reach the natural nail. Glue the crack in the natural nail and let the glue dry. Remove excess glue. Reapply the gel you beveled out and cure. Remove the sticky surface and buff the new gel flush with the remainder of the nail. Reapply a top layer of gel and cure.

Q **415. What do I do if the seal is broken and the gel has separated from the natural nail?**

A You must bevel the loose gel flush with the natural nail and reapply the gel. Be sure to wrap the gel around all sides and corners of the nails for a good seal.

Maintenance

Q **416. What is the recommended maintenance?**

A Fills are needed every two to three weeks. See the section on "Fill-ins" for more details on fills with no fill lines on pages 161–175.

Q **417. How much time should I schedule for a fill?**

A Forty-five minutes is the average.

Q **418. How often should I replace the bulbs in my UV light?**

A At least once every six months to a year.

Q **419. Do the bulbs ever burn out?**

A No, they just lose their effectiveness. In the first 3 months, the bulbs lose 30 percent of their efficiency then taper off to about 35 percent in 6 months, and at one year, they are about half as effective as they were when new.

Q *420. Which is better, shutting the light off between uses or continually leaving it on?*

A Well, turning the light on and off uses up a lot of energy. However, the life span of the bulbs if left on consistently, shortens.

Nail Notes

Nail Notes

Fill-Ins

Nail Preparation

Q *421. What do I need to do to the natural nails in preparation for an artificial overlay?*

A A series of steps to properly prepare the natural nails is important.

First have your client wash her hands before removing all polish and glue residue from repairs.

Step 1 Push the cuticles back and remove all pterygium. Do not leave any cuticle or skin attached to the nail plate. A clean, even, natural nail plate is the key to good retention. Do not shortchange this procedure. Spend ample time preparing the nails.

Step 2 Shape all ten natural nails and shorten if necessary. Shape nails square if using forms so they fit neatly under the corners of the natural nails. Shape them oval to fit the wells of the tips if you are using tips.

Step 3 Gently file the lifted product flush with the natural nail around the cuticle area. Clip if necessary, but the main goal is to remove any lifted product.

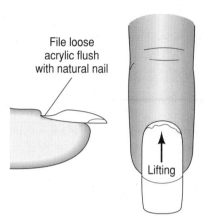

File loose
acrylic flush
with natural nail

Lifting

Removing lifted product.

Step 4 Dust nail plate with nylon brush to remove all the dust. Do not use a big fluffy brush, all you are doing is redistributing the dust from one client to another.

Step 5 Dehydrate the nail plate with a manufacturer's dehydrator. This will remove all the moisture and balance the nail.

Do not use a dehydrator when preparing for fiberglass nails. You do not want to remove the natural moisture by dehydrating the nail plate.

Step 6 Prime the nails. Two sparingly applied coats of primer is all you need. Primer application and its functions can be found on page 79.

It is also not necessary to use a primer for gels.

Q *422. I was taught to use a coarse file to rough up the natural nails before applying products. Is this not necessary?*

A The purpose of preparing the nails so carefully is to do as little damage as possible for maximum results. It is proven that gentle preparation is more effective than roughing up the natural nail. The best benefit of all is that your client doesn't need to be uncomfortable as she would be if you were roughing up the natural nail with a coarse file.

Q *423. When do I prime the nails?*

A After the dusting of the nail plate and optional use of the dehydrator.

Q *424. Can I touch the nails after I have prepared them?*

A No, you should not for two reasons. The primer may burn the skin if touched. Also, you will contaminate the nail plate and primer if you touch it, leaving oils from your skin on the nail plate which can cause lifting.

Q *425. How do I convince the client not to touch them?*

A Educate your client on your procedures by explaining what you are doing when you prepare her nails. Explain that you are removing the natural oils and dehydrating the nail plate. Ask that she not touch them or lean her hands against her face when you are working on her. She will contaminate the nails by touching her skin.

No Line Fill-Ins

The procedures in this section pertain to filling fiberglass, gels, and acrylics for a natural clear look without polish. However, these are the routine steps for a regular fill that would be polished.

Q *426. What is the procedure for fill-ins for fiberglass, gels, and acrylics?*

A There are several steps that can be used for all three products. Remember, proper nail preparation is the most crucial part of any nail service.

Step 1 Remove the polish and push cuticles back on all 10 nails.

Step 2 With a coarse file, bevel all the lifting around the cuticle area and file the product flush with the natural nail. You may want to file more than needed in order to get a truly clear fill in. Look at the profile of the nail as you file, checking to make sure you have a smooth graduation from product to natural nail. Spend as much time as needed to achieve this.

You may need to use a softer file, such as an electric file or drill using a medium or fine diamond bit. Be careful not to file too heavily into the natural nail creating a line in the natural nail plate. Gently file the exposed natural nail plate to remove any natural oils.

The trick to a clear no line fill-in is to blend the product into the natural nail without any ledges. This also makes for a strong fill-in when polishing the nails.

If you are not sure you have filed enough, apply a drop of dehydrator on the nail. The way it looks when it is wet is how it will look when it has product over it. It is kind of a sneak peek!

Step 3 For a no line fill-in, file off 25 percent of the top layer of the entire nail. This will remove any discoloration and make room for fresh product without making the nails any thicker. For a fill that you are polishing, gently buff the top of the product to rough up the surface for better adhesion.

Step 4 Reshape the parameter of all 10 nails and shorten if necessary.

Step 5 Check for stress cracks and bevel down to the natural nail through the crack. Glue the natural nail if it is broken.

Step 6 Check the sides and all edges of the tip for product separation. If the edges of the tip have separated from the natural nail, bevel the product off the edges until you reach the natural nail.

Step 7 Apply your dehydrator and primer. Prime all exposed natural nail, even the tips where you have beveled the edges. It is not necessary to prime any acrylic so apply the primer to exposed natural nail only.

Step 8 Prepare your application products.

Step 9 On all 10 nails, reapply the necessary acrylic, starting by replacing any white tip powder on the tip or in any beveled areas that have cracks.

Step 10 Next, with your pink or clear product, fill in the cuticle areas and cover the remaining nail area with fresh product.

Step 11 File all 10 nails to the desired nail shape.

Step 12 Buff all 10 nails or polish.

Q *427. Should I clip the loose or lifting products with my nippers?*

A Only if necessary. Clipping not only jars the product but leaves ledges that are not easily blended. You have to bevel the ledge flush to get a clear fill-in, causing discomfort to the client.

Q *428. What do I do if the tip of the nail is separated?*

A Bevel the loose product flush to the natural nail, exposing it. Dust it, then prime and replace the product. If you periodically do this on nails that tend to curl away naturally, you will head off the problem.

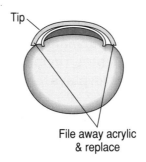

Tip

File away acrylic
& replace

Correcting the nail if the tip has separated.

Q *429. Why do the nails curl away?*

A The nails curl naturally, and when the tip product gets old, can separate. Refreshening the product will help eliminate this.

Q *430. Will filing the loose product instead of clipping it take more time?*

A Yes it will, but with practice you can conquer this procedure.

Lifting

Q *431. I am a student and I am having a lot of problems with lifting. What can I do to stop it from happening?*

A More than likely the problem is in the application of the product. Most students and inexperienced nail techs struggle when learning to work with acrylic, and application is not often smooth, especially around the cuticle and side walls, which is where the problem occurs.

Acrylic, fiberglass, and gels or any artificial product must not touch the skin and if you have applied the product so it overlaps the side wall or cuticle area, it will definitely lift. Your acrylic application should be done in smaller balls for control around these areas. The balls should be placed away from the cuticle and sidewalls, and allowed to flow smoothly to the edges without touching them. Unfortunately the perfect liquid to powder ratio plays a big factor but practice makes perfect.

There is no written rule that says the acrylic or other products have to be applied right up to the cuticle to be acceptable. A perfect graduation of product to natural nail makes for a smooth and lift-free cuticle area.

Q *432. I have several clients who have thick and hard cuticles and their nails seem to lift more than my other clients. What can I do?*

A The cuticles are the problem and need to be conditioned in order to push them back properly to prevent lifting. After each fill, you should manicure and cut her cuticles so she leaves the salon with very trim cuticles, allowing minimal growth. Do not manicure them before the fill. If you soak them before you fill them you are adding moisture to those areas that have lifted and filling them in. Have your client assist your efforts by conditioning her cuticles twice daily with the cuticle oil you recommend and retail.

There will be a noticeable difference when she returns in two weeks for her fill. Her cuticles will not be as thick, and will be softer and easier to maintain. They will also be easier to work with in preparing the nail plate for the fill. Have your client briefly wash her hands in warm water before the fill. This will soften the cuticles without soaking them. Push cuticles back, remove all the pterygium and prepare the nails for the fill.

Q *433. What is pterygium?*

A It refers to the abnormal attachment of the cuticle to the nail plate. The cuticle remains attached to the nail during its growth, thus extending out into the nail from its normal position.

Q *434. Is it necessary to remove the pterygium ?*

A Yes! This is a silent lifting culprit. Most of the time you can barely see it so it goes undetected. However, the way to tell you didn't remove all of it is if the polish does not go on smoothly at the cuticle. There is a special implement that has been designed specifically for the removal of pterygium. It's called a pterygium remover!

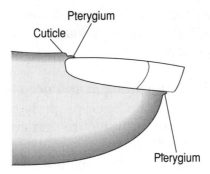

Locating the pterygium.

Q **435. Should I use a dehydrator before I apply the acrylic to prevent lifting?**

A Removing oils and moisture when preparing the natural nail for any artificial service is a must, and part of the procedure may include a dehydrator. Some manufacturers recommend one with their line to enhance the retention of the artificial products. However, you must read the labels of these products to identify any kind of alcohol in the contents. Alcohol has an oily base to it and can hurt the retention of the acrylic by replacing oils you just removed. A white chalky appearance after the dehydrator dries will let you know it is ready to receive primer. Also, you do not want to use a dehydrator with fiberglass nails.

Any shiny areas left on the natural nail are spots that contain oils that were missed.

Q **436. Sometimes I get a pocket in the middle of the acrylic nail that has lifted. What causes this and how do I fix it?**

A The product has become brittle or the client has somehow jarred the acrylic in the center of her nail, sometimes without even knowing it. I have found that some acrylic products are more susceptible to this than others and by switching to one that works better for you, you can solve the problem.

To fix the lifting in the center, file the top of the loose acrylic until you make a hole, exposing the natural nail. Continue to file the loose acrylic on the edges of the hole flush with the natural nail until there is no lifted acrylic left. Prime the exposed natural nail and reapply acrylic.

Q **437. The tips of my client's natural nails seem to lift away from the acrylic. Why does this happen and how can I prevent it from happening again?**

A The acrylic at the tip has become old and brittle and has broken down the retention between the natural nail and acrylic. This is usually due to the fact that this nail has not been replaced in a while, and you might consider replacing it now. This will happen more to clients who are gentle with their nails and don't break them often.

Tip maintenance should be part of a regular fill. Ignoring the tips can result in separation. If the tip comes loose, file down the acrylic on each corner edge of the tip until you expose the natural nail that has separated. Prime the exposed natural nail and refill the corners with acrylic.

Clients who have natural nails that tend to curl seem to have this problem more frequently. Wearing the nail square instead of round can also help. Periodically touching up the underneath with glue can also prevent the separation.

Q **438. I have a client who has very sweaty hands, and I cannot get her nails to stay down no matter what product I use or how many times I prime the nails. What do I do?**

A Not all clients are created equal, and not all can wear artificial nails. Trying different products and techniques is not always the answer so let's take the business approach.

Let's say hypothetically she gets her nails filled every two weeks. Her fill takes over an hour because she lifts so badly and there is so much repair work to do. This client seems to be a 1 week fill client, so advise her that a weekly fill will allow you to head off any problems so she can comfortably wear her nails without lifting. Charge her a special weekly fill price and let her know that your commitment to solving her problems is as important as her spending a little more time in the salon. With a weekly fill, your fill time with her should be considerably less because you are doing less work.

Q *439. If a client has a nail that has lifted and cannot get it fixed right away, what do I suggest to the client?*

A Nail glue is the best temporary remedy until the client can get her nail repaired. Instruct the client to make sure the nail is dry before applying the glue. The smaller the amount of glue the better the bond. More is not necessarily better. Tell her to drop a bit of glue on the crack and hold the crack open a bit so the glue seeps in. Then squeeze the crack closed and let dry. Buff the glue smooth and repolish. Another temporary solution is a vinyl mender that comes under several names and is sold by several companies, the most common being Crack Attack. Placed on top of polish, it will seal the crack temporarily without the need for glue. It is easily removed and is acetone resistant.

Q *440. Does taking medication affect lifting?*

A Yes. Cold pills, antihistamines, large doses of B-6, heart medicine, and medication for diabetics can cause lifting by drying out the skin and nails. Using lotion and cuticle oil is your best attack in preventing dry skin.

Q *441. Does the weather affect lifting?*

A Yes. The winter seems to dry out the nails, cuticle, and skin, causing brittleness and lifting. The condition of the hands and nails from harsh and cold climates can be devastating to a nail technician's business. The heat causes the nails and skin to produce more oils, especially if it gets hot fast, as it does in desert areas.

Q *442. The acrylic line I use claims that I don't need to use primer. Is this true?*

A In some cases, with some clients, no matter what you put on their nails they won't lift. With these clients, you don't need to use a primer because it is not necessary. However, on the average client, you need primer.

Backfills

Q *443. What is a backfill?*

A A backfill is when you replace the white acrylic on the tip of a pink and white sculptured nail or an acrylic tip and overlay. This is an added technique in the fill-in procedure.

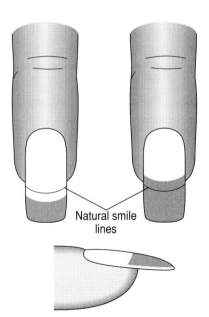

Natural smile
lines

A backfill. 1: The shaded area represents white tip powder; 2: Cut out the shaded area. Remove 75% of the white tip acrylic powder

Q 444. Who gets a backfill?

A The client who wears acrylic nails with the permanent French manicure look, which is pink or clear, and white tip powders usually without polish or a clear top coat.

Q 445. Do you charge more for a backfill?

A Yes, you should. Add $5 to $10 to the regular fill price for backfills. Not only are you offering a more labor intensive service, you are using more products and offering new techniques.

Q 446. How often do you need to do a backfill?

A Depends on how high you place the white tip smile line when applying the white tip product and how fast the client's nails grow. You can make them last from 1 fill or up to three, but the average is to do a backfill every other or every third fill-in appointment.

Q 447. Does a backfill take more time?

A Yes, it does and practice makes perfect. At first it will take you approximately 15 to 30 extra minutes. Until you get this service to fit into your regular fill-in schedule you should allow more time.

Q 448. What do I use for a backfill?

A An electric file or drill is usually used to do a backfill. However this can be done with a hand file.

Q *449. What are the benefits of backfilling?*

A It gives the client a permanent French manicure look that is polish free. There is no waiting for the polish to dry. It provides the client with a special service that allows her to have "fresh" or "brand new" looking nails every time she visits the salon.

Q *450. What are the procedures for a backfill?*

A First you must follow the steps on "No Line Fills" in the previous section. Then:

Step 1 After you have prepared the cuticle area and other lifted areas, reshape and shorten the nails if necessary.

Step 2 File the entire top of the acrylic nail removing the top layer of discoloration.

Step 3 Starting on the right side of the smile line, at an angle, cut into the nail where you want the new smile line to

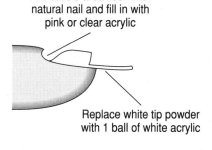

File cuticle area flush with
natural nail and fill in with
pink or clear acrylic

Replace white tip powder
with 1 ball of white acrylic

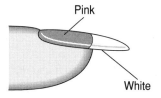

Pink

White

Finished Nail

Procedures for a backfill.

be. Cut a "U" shape that is similar to the shape of the cuticle across the nail to the other side where the smile line ends. The beveling should cut into the nail only about 75 percent, never touching the natural nail. You have just beveled a new smile line in the nail.

Step 4 Holding the nail so you can see the profile of the entire nail, place the bit flat on the remaining white tip product and remove approximately 75 percent.

Step 5 After you have removed 75 percent of the white tip, dust the nail again.

Step 6 Prime the exposed natural nail around the cuticle and any spots on the tip that may be exposed. Do not prime the white acrylic tip left on the tips of the nail, because it will cause yellowing.

Step 7 Apply the new white tip powder to all ten nails. Start by placing 1 medium size ball of white acrylic in the center of the tip and up against the beveled smile line. Wipe your brush, pat the product to the left and to the right, and then wipe it down to the edge of the tip.

Look at the nail from the side view and make sure that the white tip powder is taller than the pink or clear on the base of the nail. The reason for applying all ten white tips first is so you don't interchange the white powder and the pink or clear powder. Another reason is that you allow the white tip to dry before applying the pink or clear over it, so you don't drag the pink or clear through the wet white tip.

Step 8 If needed, add a small amount to each "ear" of the smile line for maximum coverage.

Step 9 After you have completed the white tip application wipe your brush clean and use fresh liquid for the pink or clear application. Otherwise your product will look cloudy.

Step 10 Fill in the cuticle areas and extend fresh pink or clear product to the new smile line coating the entire nail with fresh product.

Q 451. What drill bits should I use for the backfill?

A For the cleanest and quickest cuts, use a small carbide bit or a medium diamond bit. A cardboard disposable bit doesn't cut as clean. Refer to section "Backfill Bits" on page 181.

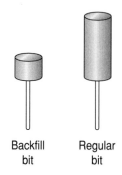

Backfill
bit

Regular
bit

A backfill drill bit and regular bit.

Nail Notes

Drills & Electric Files

Proper Use of the Drill

Q *452. Is a drill and an electric file the same thing?*

A It depends on the manufacturer's or technician's choice of terminology but they are basically the same tool.

Q *453. What is the biggest misconception about using drills?*

A That they are dangerous. They are not dangerous. Only the operator using them is dangerous when the drill is not used correctly.

Q *454. Can drills really be used safely?*

A Yes, with the proper education a drill or electric file can be as safe as a file.

Q *455. Are drills really faster?*

A They can be when the nails are sculpted well and the drill is used properly. However, filing can be as quick in the same circumstance.

Q 456. How can I learn how to use the drill before I actually use it on a client?

A Practice on yourself and take a manufacturer's class on the proper use of a drill. Break in your drill bit so that it is not as sharp, or use a used one first to practice.

Q 457. What speeds do drills come in?

A That depends of the drill. Usually a drill will have a variety of speeds to choose from.

Q 458. What is RPM?

A Revolutions per minute; in other words, the speed.

Q 459. Can a left-handed technician use a drill?

A Yes, if it has a reverse mode.

Q 460. What is the shank?

A This is the size of the neck of the drill bit.

Q 461. What sizes does the shank come in?

A There are two basic sizes: 1/8" and 3/32".

Q *462. What are the types of bits available?*

A There are three basic types of bits, carbides, diamond bits, and sanders that all come in a variety of sizes:

Barrel
Small Barrel
Cone
Football
Sander
2 Week Backfill
4 Week Backfill
Chamois Buffers

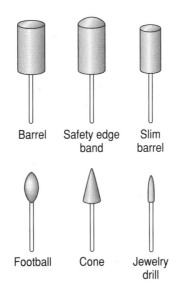

| Barrel | Safety edge band | Slim barrel |

| Football | Cone | Jewelry drill |

Various bit shapes.

Q *463. What is a carbide bit?*

A A carbide bit is a bit made of high carbide alloy of stainless steel. Diamond, cross, or single cut designs are machined into the bit for cutting purposes. A carbide bit shaves the surface of the nails instead of vibrating it off like a diamond bit or file.

Q 464. What is a diamond bit?

A It has diamond-like specks of product on the outside edges of the bit.

Q 465. What grits do the diamond and sander bits come in?

A Coarse, medium, and fine.

Q 466. How do I keep the heat from the drill down?

A Proper use of the drill requires regularly taking the bit off the nail as you are working to alleviate any heating of the nail.

Q 467. How do I clean the bits?

A You can safely soak them in acetone to remove any acrylic product that may get stuck.

Q 468. Should I sanitize the bits?

A Yes, you should, just like you would the implements. After soaking them in acetone, rinse them with soap and water and sanitize them in sanitation solution.

Q 469. How do I clean the drill?

A Leave the cleaning and maintenance to the manufac- turer. The casing on the drill should protect it from dust and you should periodically wipe the case off with a damp cloth.

Q *470. What do I need to do if I am having problems with my drill?*

A Call your manufacturer and follow their instructions.

Backfill Bits

Q *471. What is the best bit to use for a backfill?*

A A diamond or carbide bit is the best for a backfill.

Q *472. Can I use a sander band bit?*

A Yes, but they are not as smooth as a carbide or diamond bit.

Q *473. How does the backfill bit work?*

A Because it is short, it will cut into the smile line area only. All you have to do is fill in the new smile line with a matching white tip product.

Q *474. Why do the backfill bits come in two sizes?*

A One is for two week's growth and the other is for three to four week's growth.

Q 475. Do the backfill bits come in different grits and types?

A Yes, you can find carbides, diamond, and sander bits in all three grits: coarse, medium, and fine.

Equipment

Q 476. What equipment do you need to operate a drill?

A This depends on the way you want to set up your drill. If you want to mount it on your station, you will need brackets, screws, and a screwdriver.

Q 477. Do all drills come with a foot pedal?

A Foot pedals are optional and do not come with all drills or electric files. If you choose to purchase a drill with a foot pedal, the benefit is that you can change the speed of the drill as you use it, never having to stop. If you use a drill without a foot pedal, you can choose the desired speed before you use the drill. If you need to adjust the speed, you need to stop and do so.

Q 478. What do I do with the drill handle when it is not in use?

A A stand usually made from rubber or metal should accompany your drill.

Q 479. Is there any other equipment needed to operate a drill?

A No, they are pretty simple and easy to set up for use.

Nail Notes

Polish

Application Techniques

Q 480. What should I do to prepare the nails for polishing?

A A squeaky clean nail plate is most important for good polish adhesion. There should be no cuticle skin on the nail plate, and all foreign matter must be removed.

Q 481. What should I use to clean the nail plate?

A Soap and water is best for cleaning a clean nail plate. Acetone and alcohol have an oily base and can leave residue on the nail plate, making the polish wobble and not stick to the sides of the nail as well.

Q 482. What kind of base coat is the best for natural nails?

A A thin base coat that dries almost instantly is the best for use on natural nails. It provides a good surface to polish and protects the natural nails from absorbing the color. It also makes for easy polish removal.

Q *483. Should I use a base coat under a liquid wrap?*

A This is not necessary since most liquid wraps are a neutral color and can act as a base coat. Liquid wraps are thicker than regular polish and another unnecessary coat of polish will only slow down the drying process.

Q *484. How can I get the polish to dry faster?*

A Thin applications with time to dry between each coat can help.

Q *485. Should I shake the polish before polishing?*

A You can, but it may cause air bubbles. Have the client choose her color before starting her service and shake the bottle of polish then. The polish will settle during the manicure.

Step 1 Before you apply the polish, swirl the neck of the brush inside the neck of the bottle as you slowly work the brush

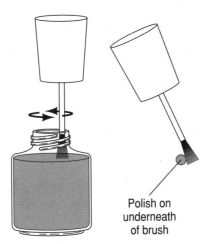

Polish on
underneath
of brush

Before applying polish, swirl the neck of the brush inside the neck of the bottle while slowly removing the brush from the bottle.

out of the bottle. As the brush leaves the top of the bottle, wipe the side of the brush furthest away from you pressing the polish to one side of the brush. This gives you better control of the polish in the brush.

Step 2 Place a drop of polish in the center of the nail just below the cuticle and polish downward to the tip of the nail. Take the brush and place another drop of polish on the left side of the nail, a little lower than the first one, right under the cuticle, and polish downward. Then place a third drop of polish on the right side and polish downward. Take the remainder of the polish and wipe the edge of the tip. The perfect nail should be polished in three sections with one application of polish.

Not all nails are the same and some may need a second dip into the bottle for complete coverage. Some nails are longer than others and also need extra polish.

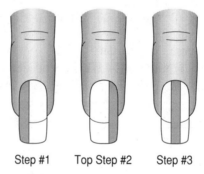

Step #1   Top Step #2   Step #3

Three steps for applying polish.

Q **486. What is the best tool to use for cleaning up the polish?**

A A polish corrector pen dipped in acetone is the best but an orangewood stick can also be effective. A size 4 sculpting brush with a perfect point is also a great tool for clean up. Dip the brush sparingly into acetone, then take the brush around the polished cuticle area for a perfectly smooth look.

Top Coats

Q 487. *What is a top coat?*

A It is the final sealer which is applied over the base coat and usually two coats of color. Its purpose is to strengthen and protect the color.

Q 488. *Are all top coats the same?*

A No, they are not. The chemical makeup is similar but the actual final product can be different from company to company. Quality, viscosity, drying time, hardeners, and sunscreens are all variations that can be found in different top coats.

Q 489. *What about light-cured fast-setting top coats?*

A These are the perfect top coats for polished nails that have an artificial surface to them. Drying time is anywhere from 60 seconds to 3 minutes. A special base coat must be used on natural nails in order to get the same results in drying and protection.

Q 490. *Can any top coat be used with a UV light?*

A Although it is probably not recommended by manufacturers, it can be done with very successful results.

Q 491. *Should you use a different top coat on natural nails?*

A There are special natural nail topcoats or ones that are formulated just for natural nails that can enhance the longevity of the polish.

Q 492. Do all top coats have sunscreen?

A No, they don't. Most will and they usually advertise it on the bottle.

Q 493. What are plasticizer top coats?

A Plastic coatings that are applied like a top coat that contain ultraviolet inhibitors. You cannot polish on top or underneath them, and they cannot be removed with polish remover or acetone. Buffing is the only way to remove them, or they can safely be filled over without removing.

Troubleshooting

Q 494. My clients move and don't pay attention when I polish which causes me to make mistakes. What can I do?

A Preparing your client for the polish is your responsibility, so have them pay and get their keys out. Then ask that they help you polish by paying attention. Explain that you have a schedule to keep and you cannot fix any spoiled polish jobs.

Q 495. I have trouble with air bubbles in my polish. What causes them?

A Air bubbles are caused by the disruption of the polish as in shaking. Humidity can also cause air bubbles.

Q 496. The tips of the polish always rub off. Is there anything I can do to prevent this from happening?

A Cover the edge of the tip with an ample amount of top coat to protect the color from wearing. The clear top coat will wear off first. A trick to this is to apply a top coat every night after the manicure. Don't wait until the polish starts to wear. Protect it before it starts to wear off.

Q 497. Why does the polish on my French manicures turn yellow?

A Mostly because the top coat does not have ultraviolet inhibitors in it. The sunscreen lotion you use at the beach will also yellow polish.

Q 498. Why does my polish dent hours after it was done?

A The polish has not completely dried underneath and needs to dry a little between applications of each coat of polish.

Q 499. How long does polish take to completely dry?

A It can take up to 8 hours to completely cure.

Q 500. How can I avoid sheet marks in my polish from sleeping?

A This is the same reason they dent; the polish is not completely cured and is not completely dry. Allowing each coat of polish to dry between applications can help dry the polish.

Q 501. How do I prevent my polish from getting thick?

A Exposure to the air when you are polishing will thicken the polish that is in the bottle. A thinner or a drop of acetone will thin polish to the desired consistency.

Q 502. What do I do if the polish is too thin and doesn't cover the nails well?

A Three coats may be necessary. Leave the bottle open for a while and allow it to thicken. The more you use it, the thicker it will get.

Nail Notes

Etc. . .

The Right Brush

Q *503. Why is a brush so important?*

A You can't build good nails without good tools. Your brush is your most important tool and should be kept in perfect condition at all times.

Q *504. What kind of a brush should I use for sculpting?*

A A sable brush of your choice. A sable brush is usually made from the finest quality hairs, and provides good application and workability. The tip of the brush is a perfect shape, hairs never fall out, and the brush will last a long time. Usually, the cheaper the brush, the cheaper the quality. You will find that the hairs don't stay together well and are of different lengths, and the workability is not as good.

Q *505. What shape brush should I be using to apply acrylic?*

A A pointed brush is the most popular, an oval the second, and a flat square brush is the least popular.

Q 506. What size brushes are the most frequently used?

A Sizes 6 and 7 are the most popular. Size 8 is for the seasoned tech and sizes 4 or 5 for the sculptor using smaller amounts of acrylic balls.

Q 507. Do I need to clean my brush periodically?

A Always wipe your brush clean with leftover liquid after using it and never put it away with dried acrylic in it. This will eliminate the need to use brush cleaners on a regular basis.

Q 508. Can I use acetone to clean my brush?

A Acetone is extremely harsh on your brush and you should not use it unless necessary. Remember fur coats are made of sable hair and they aren't cleaned with acetone.

Q 509. How often do I need to replace my brush?

A Every few months is the norm. A good brush should last for at least that and a cheaper one less.

Q 510. How much should I pay for a sculpting brush?

A Approximately $12 to $15 is the average cost of a good sculpting brush.

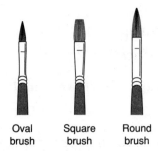

Oval brush   Square brush   Round brush

Various brush shapes.

The Benefits of Using Systems

Q *511. What is a system?*

A A system is the complete product line from one company that when used as the manufacturer suggests, will give you the maximum results.

Q *512. How do I as a nail technician benefit from using a system?*

A Each product line is formulated and designed to work together harmoniously, providing good results and wearability for the client.

Q *513. Can I safely mix products in different systems?*

A Depends on the products. Cuticle oils, lotions, sanitation products, dehydrators, and primers can be interchangeable. However, the manufacturers who make these, products will not guarantee them if not used with the complete system.

Q *514. Can I safely use a liquid from one system and a powder from another?*

A This is not advisable. Chemicals within these products can interchange and cause allergic reactions to the clients as well as application and durability problems. For example, the catalyst may be in the liquid of one product and the powder of the other. You could end up using a product that has no catalyst at all, and by mixing liquids and powders, develop a reaction. We are not chemists and should not play with chemicals. Each product, although similar, can be very different.

Product Contamination

Q 515. *How does one contaminate products?*

A By not understanding contamination. For instance, if your nippers are submerged below the liquid line of your sanitation solution, how do you retrieve the nippers? With your fingers that have nail dust and cuticle oil on them? Or do you use a sanitized tong every time? Do you place the tong in a sanitary container between use? If not, you are contaminating your sanitation solution. Sometimes our daily habits become so routine that we don't even know we are contaminating our products.

Q 516. *How do you know if you have contaminated a product?*

A If it appears cloudy and has dust-like particles in the bottom of the container. For example, look at your primer bottle. Is there nail dust in the bottom?

Q 517. *Should I use a separate brush for each liquid and powder system I use?*

A Yes, if you don't, you are marrying your products.

Q 518. *How can I avoid contaminating my acrylic liquid?*

A Pour only as much as you need for the current client into your dappan dish. Dispose of the leftover and do not pour it back into the original bottle. Do not work directly out of the bottle, and if you use a pump, use the ones with the mushroom top that keep the liquid from backwashing into the container.

Q *519. How can I avoid contaminating my primer and dehydrators?*

A Use a smaller applicator bottle and pour enough for one week's use into it. Wipe the bottle out at the end of the week and start with fresh product every week.

Q *520. How can I avoid contaminating my sculpting brush?*

A Never, never, never touch it with your fingers. Wipe with leftover liquid and put away.

Timing

Q *521. How long should it take me to do a manicure?*

A One half hour to 45 minutes is the average.

Q *522. How long should I be spending for a pedicure?*

A One hour.

Q *523. How long should I schedule for a full set of nails?*

A One to 1-1/2 hours.

Here is a guideline for a 1 hr. and 15 minute full set:

15 minutes to prepare the nails
30 minutes for application of sculptured nails
15 minutes to apply tips
20 minutes to apply overlays

15 minutes for filing
10 minutes for buffing
10 minutes for polishing

Q *524. What is the average time for a fill?*

A One hour or less.

Here is a guideline for a 60-minute fill.

5 minutes to remove polish
10 minutes for nail preparation
10–15 minutes for application
10 minutes filing and shaping
5 minutes buffing and finishing
5–6 minutes washing hands and nails
1 minute for paying
5–8 minutes for polishing or high shine buffing

Nail Removal

Q *525. How does one remove artificial nails?*

A Soaking the nails in acetone, non-acetone, or nail remover products will melt the nail off.

Q *526. What should the client soak in?*

A A glass bowl is the best. A plastic manicure bowl will melt if using acetone.

Q *527. How long does soaking take?*

A Depending on the thickness of the acrylic, up to 45 minutes. If the client submerges her nails fully for 45 minutes, they should fall right off.

Q **528. What is the procedure for removing the artificial nails?**

A After soaking for 30 minutes or so, you may want to remove the nails one hand at a time. Take a paper towel and gently wipe off the product that has melted to a soft state. Replace the nails in the remover right away and remove the other hand. The acrylic will start to set up again as soon as you remove it from the acetone or remover.

While soaking, you may want to cover the bowl with a towel so the client doesn't have to smell the acetone or remover.

Q **529. Does it cause any damage to the natural nail?**

A No, but you may want to condition the nails and cuticles after this treatment. As a precaution, you may want to cover the cuticles with petroleum jelly to protect them while soaking.

Q **530. Can you soak gels off in these products?**

A The newer gels on the market can be softened with acetone and nail remover, and can be peeled off when soft.

Q **531. What are the other alternatives to removing nails?**

A Clipping them off is the most dangerous to the nail plate and totally unnecessary. Filing them off is a more effective alternative but can be quite uncomfortable.

Q **532. Can I also soak fiberglass silk, or paper wraps off this way?**

A Yes, and in less time than it takes for an acrylic to soak off.

Nail Notes

Appendix

Bibliography

Milady Publishing Company. *Milady's Art and Science of Nail Technology*. Albany: Milady Publishing Company, 1992.

Nails Magazine. "How to Read Your MSDS." *Nails 1995 Fact Book*. Redondo Beach: Bobit Publishing Company, 1995: 14–28.

Owens, Barbara. "Brush Strokes." *NailPro Magazine*, July 1995: 34–39.

Peters, Vicki. "Fiberglass Basics." *NailPro Magazine*, December 1994: 22–28.

Peters, Vicki. "All the Angles." *NailPro Magazine*, April 1995: 32–41.

Peters, Vicki. "Sculpting Pink and White." *NailPro, Magazine*, May 1995: 32–41.

Peters, Vicki. "Disinfection Dialog." *NailPro Magazine*, June 1995: 46–52, 134.

Peters, Vicki. "Building Speed." *NailPro Magazine*, July 1995: 40–48.

Peters, Vicki. "Versatile Gels." *NailPro Magazine*, August 1995: 64–70.

Peters, Vicki. "Fitting Forms." *NailPro Magazine*, September 1995: 28–32.

Schoon, Douglas. *HIV/AIDS and Hepatitis: Everything You Need to Know to Protect Yourself and Others*. Albany: Milady Publishing Company, 1994.

Glossary/Index